To my wife, who taught me how to give

To my children, the greatest of gifts

CONTENTS

INTRODUCTION **How I Discovered the Hidden Core** 1

CHAPTER 1 **The Brain and the Spine:**
Fix It Even If It Ain't Broke 11

CHAPTER 2 **Pain** 27

CHAPTER 3 **The Anomaly and Anatomy of the Back** 59

CHAPTER 4 **The Hidden Core Workout** 83

CHAPTER 5 **Diagnosis: A DIY Guide** 121

CHAPTER 6 **The Nonsurgical Treatment of Back Pain** 157

CHAPTER 7 **Surgery** 183

CHAPTER 8 **The Back Genome** 211

ACKNOWLEDGMENTS 227

NOTES 229

INDEX 233

ABOUT THE AUTHOR 245

HOW I DISCOVERED
THE HIDDEN CORE

I T WAS ONE of those experiences you don't forget. Many years ago, when I was a neurosurgery resident, I was awakened in the middle of the night by a call from a new patient named Tom.

"If I had a gun," he said, "I would blow my brains out."

My heart pounded as I tried to figure out how to respond. All I could think to do was ask the simplest, most obvious question: "What's wrong?" The floodgates opened. Tom told me he was suffering from excruciating pain in his back. He had sought help from various providers over the years, he said, but nothing was working. His pain just kept getting worse, and finally, in his bleakest moments alone, the pain had reached a debilitating level. His back pain was so severe that he was unable to move. He was sure that he needed surgery, and feared lifelong disability.

After listening to Tom, I tried to dispel his darkest fears by explaining to him what was happening—why his back likely hurt and what might happen over the coming days. I suspected that most of his pain was the result of muscle spasm. I assured him that as painful as this episode was, it was a common occurrence that would subside within a day or two. I provided Tom with a plan, complete with a timetable of when to expect to feel some relief.

I was curious as to whether the pain he was experiencing had changed now that his fear had decreased and his anxiety was under control. "Do you need some medication for the pain tonight?" I asked.

"Doc," Tom said, "I have to tell you the strangest thing. At this moment, I have no pain at all."

Later that night, awake in bed, I was struck by this question: In a matter of minutes, how could Tom go from experiencing pain that made him suicidal to experiencing no pain at all? The encounter planted a seed in my mind that would ultimately grow into a deep interest in back pain. But my interest has other sources as well, some of them more personal.

When I was a teenager, my father bought a Roman chair and put it into the basement to complete his primitive home gym. Sometimes referred to as a hyperextension machine, a Roman chair looks like a cross between a pommel horse and a prayer kneeler. It's designed to work the muscles in your back and abdomen and is usually positioned in a gym near the pull-up bars or any other piece of equipment built to pit you against your own body weight.

I used to use the chair in high school, particularly when my back acted up, which happened more often than I wanted to admit. Because I was active in sports, my back frequently gave me fits. The morning after a game, for instance, I could sometimes barely put on my shoes. I had to learn how to slip them on without bending over or using my hands.

No one *recommended* the Roman chair for my back pain; I discovered its usefulness quite by chance. With the innocent curiosity of a young

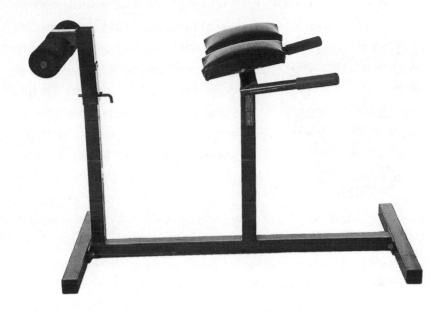

person, I experimented with my father's device, and I was surprised to discover that my back immediately felt better. I didn't understand *why* it helped, but I remember going down to the basement and using it whenever my back hurt, even during an acute episode of pain. I'm certain that if this chair had not been introduced to me early in life, I would have learned either to rest or to resist exercise during an acute episode of pain.

Fast-forward twenty years to my late thirties. (Believe me, it feels like time went that fast!) I was at a party and met a man named Jake. He had heard that I was a neurosurgeon and couldn't wait to tell me how he'd overcome his own back pain, which had been crippling. He had tried epidural injections, physical therapy, chiropractic, and acupuncture—all without success. In frustration, he had searched the Internet and ultimately connected with the world of kettlebells—cast-iron cannonball-shaped weights with handles.

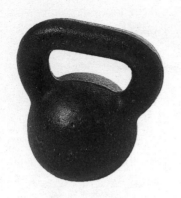

Over a period of months he had strengthened his body by swinging the kettlebells. He started to notice two things: His back felt better, and he felt fitter than ever before. He was in his fifties and had recently entered and won an international strength competition for his age and weight class. (Admittedly, there aren't a lot of fifty-year-olds who weigh 140 pounds and want to compete in such an event.)

As he spoke, I was mesmerized. How could a guy in his fifties make such a transition? How did he have the nerve to pursue such a vigorous program with debilitating back pain? But then I remembered my own experience as a teenager and, later, as a newly minted neurosurgeon, when I, too, had discovered that exercising, even while in pain, had met with success.

When I was just starting to practice neurosurgery, I experienced a month-long episode of severe back pain. A magnetic resonance imaging (MRI) test of my lumbar spine revealed a herniated L5–S1 disc, as well as a chronic condition called spondylolisthesis—the result of a stress fracture that had occurred while I was playing football years before (and that undoubtedly had been the cause of my adolescent back pain). I showed my MRI to my neurosurgical peers, who uniformly recommended surgery. I was just starting my career, however, and couldn't bear the idea of spending several weeks in recovery.

Although I had always preached the importance of exercise to my patients, I was too frightened to undertake any exertion myself. My pain had improved enough for me to function, but the fear that exercise would bring it back prevented me from following my own advice. Slowly, though, my hypocrisy ate away at me, until I finally got up and, despite the pain, started to exercise. I returned to the Roman chair. I started slowly, with a few reps, then steadily increased the intensity of my workouts. I felt an immediate difference. My back began to feel a comforting sense of tone and strength. As my back pain slowly receded, I became convinced that I was on the right track.

Years later, while I was listening to Jake, all of these thoughts came together. In each case an active approach to exercise had helped alleviate back pain. I didn't quite know it yet, but I had just backed my way into discovering the importance of strengthening the back muscles and the correlation between these muscles and back pain, both as a *cause* and as a *solution*. I also realized that this kind of exercise could be initiated earlier than is traditionally accepted in the course of a patient's treatment.

My search of the literature revealed similar explorations into exercise strategies, but the strategies described had only sporadic success and thus had never become mainstream. That research convinced me that pain-plagued back muscles could be exercised safely, however, and so I began to treat my more ambitious patients with intense backstrengthening. The patients who committed to the program were rewarded with terrific results.

CORE CONSIDERATIONS

The muscles of the back—particularly the multifidus muscles—are an integral part of our "core," but they have too often been overlooked. I like to think of these muscles as the body's "hidden core." Our culture has experienced a rich history of strengthening the core to alleviate back pain, a history that peaked in the 1990s when the transversalis muscle (the deep muscle located in the front of your abdomen) was singled out as the essence of the core. This faulty and incomplete definition of "core" suggested that an isolated group of muscles could be developed and used to stabilize the spine and, in turn, reduce back pain. The discipline of Pilates, for example, promotes the strengthening of the transversalis muscle as a means to stabilize the trunk of the body during movement, which limits stress on the spine.

While this movement has met with some success, it hasn't turned out to be the panacea that was hoped for in its initial stages. Isolating the front of the core is only half the story, and studies have shown that it can cause an asymmetry that may even weaken the back,[1] an outcome that I will explain later in the book. By contrast, the approach outlined in this book focuses on continuing the strengthening program *around* the entire back—the front, the sides, and the back—like a brace, or the body's natural weight-lifting belt.

Most of us design our exercise programs after a perusal of our appearance in the mirror. We want better abdominal muscles, better pectorals, and better biceps. Strengthening the abdominal muscles may be the brass ring if you want to be the newest cast member of a reality TV show. The key to back health, however, is to focus on muscles that can't be seen in the mirror. Through this new paradoxical and effective approach to strengthening your core, the exercises of the Hidden Core Workout will help you treat your back pain once and for all. Oh, and you might even look great in the process!

This approach stems from a need to attend to my own debilitating back pain as well as from my studies, specialization, and experience as chief of neurosurgery—as a neurosurgeon who prefers to offer his patients an effective workout before offering them a scalpel.

What *The End of Back Pain* does that other books on back pain do not is provide plenty of *rational information* about pain, your reaction to it, your perception of it, and your innate ability to be a person of action, *especially* when in pain. It provides a prescriptive and *systematic approach* to alleviating back pain, while simultaneously changing how you think about back pain. I'm going to engage not only your body, but also your intellect. This is why you will find sprinkled throughout the book some thoughts from famous philosophers. You might think it a little odd for a book about back pain to invoke Nietzsche, Descartes, Kierkegaard, and Sartre. But it turns out that these thinkers have a lot to teach us about the psychological, physiological, and emotional driving forces of back pain.

In the following pages, you'll find out how to change your mindset from the passive and punitive ("What's wrong with me?") to the actionable and attainable ("What do I need to do to improve my function?") and, at the same time, fulfill your personal quest for living with less pain.

Over the past twenty-five years, I have seen patients who, like Tom, feel hopeless and helpless because of debilitating, depressing, and disruptive chronic or acute back pain. Perhaps your back pain, too, has led you down a proverbial rabbit hole of inconsistent or contradicting diagnoses, alternative therapies, pain medications, unnecessary surgeries, and even desperation. I understand the physical and emotional effects this particular type of pain can have on a person, especially when the source of the pain is unknown.

Back pain is not the problem. How we *deal* with back pain is. While a sobering 80 percent of us will suffer from back pain at some point—and nearly 50 percent of us have experienced back pain in the past year!—treatment for back pain has been found largely ineffective when scrutinized by modern, evidence-based medicine.

FREEDOM, AND FREEDOM FROM PAIN

Throughout this book, I will suggest that the solution to this problem involves a transition from the current system, which treats back pain in a way that's paternalistically driven, to a system that puts the patient in the driver's seat so that he or she is actively involved in the "promotion of health" as opposed to being passively subjected to the "treatment of disease." In this new system, the patient is directed to maximize function as opposed to minimize pain.

The English philosopher Francis Bacon famously said, "Knowledge is power." We need to disabuse ourselves first and foremost of how we currently define pain and react to it, and replace this with knowledge that will serve to mitigate pain. Tom's pain, for instance, was alleviated when I was able to offer him a clear picture of what was happening to him and where to go from there.

For you, we'll begin "powering up" with some new insights and knowledge about back pain. Like Tom, once you're less afraid of how you feel and what you feel, you can begin to calm yourself and focus on forging a path to the core solution—using that hidden core I mentioned earlier. These insights and knowledge will introduce you to the power of independence. Although this book sets out to provide effective techniques for managing your back pain, its larger and overarching goal is to liberate you, not just from pain, but from dependence on others.

Back pain is an unfortunate part of life. Setbacks and unexpected flare-ups will predictably occur. The goal for any patient with back pain is not to eliminate pain totally, but to change your body in such a way as to minimize the pain and its effect on you. Regardless of the cause of your pain, you can almost always reduce its intensity, its duration, and its frequency of occurrence. Understanding and accepting back pain as a part of life, instead of chasing your tail in the search of a nonexistent cure-all to pain, lets you instead expend your energy on increasing function. The good news is this reduction in setbacks can almost always be accomplished with the Hidden Core Workout.

I have woven a series of paradoxes throughout this book, which I refer to as "hidden truths." These are designed to disrupt your status quo and to remind you that this book is as much about *un*learning as it is about learning. Not only will you learn that "your back should be straight when it's bent" and that "pain medication causes pain," you will also figure out an approach to back pain, both novel and optimistic, with help from ancient philosophers and several cutting-edge doctrines of modern psychology.

This is not a book about labeling your back pain; it's about learning not to be preoccupied or overwhelmed by that pain and to do what you might never have done before—exercise the hidden core.

CHAPTER 1

THE BRAIN AND THE SPINE

FIX IT EVEN IF IT AIN'T BROKE

Picture yourself as a fifty-year-old man who recently had a minor heart attack. What would you do? How would you live?

I'll bet that you would feel frightened and vulnerable. You would be motivated by that fear to follow your doctor's advice. You might also pray that the medications that reduce inflammation, blood pressure, and cholesterol would protect your heart. You would likely modify your diet and exercise habits (at least temporarily).

Sadly, you would likely accept that you've been cursed with a "bad" heart and hope that today's high-tech medical system could come to your rescue and keep you ticking.

Alternatively, how many of you, after that minor heart attack, would methodically train for, and begin running, marathons? How many of you would radically change the way you eat and, say, become a vegan? How many of you would reduce your body weight down to your weight at age eighteen? How many of you would *not* accept that you've been cursed with a "bad" heart, but rather set out to *change* your heart? How many of you think that you could actually change the size and flow of your coronary arteries?

You can. You can also change your back—for the better.

THE "ANTIFRAGILE" BACK

This book is about changing your back.

Before your back can be changed, however, your mind must be changed. The very activities that you imagine will make your back hurt can make your back stronger—and fundamentally different.

The transformation of both your back and your mind can be accomplished by leveraging the almost magical synergy that exists between the brain and the body.

That transformation also takes advantage of our (and many other creatures') innate capacity to change in response to stress or any other factor that disrupts our equilibrium. As an example of that capacity, when groups of rats are placed in two different environments, the brains of those in the more varied and challenging environment flourish more.[1]

Conventional wisdom views stress (and resulting inflammation) as the foundation of disease and aging. Rather than viewing stress as eroding or weakening, however, we can and should welcome it as a source of growth and health. Stress has a "sweet spot," however. Too much, and we will be weakened; too little, and we will fail to grow and attain health. Stress also needs to be coupled with adequate "recovery" periods to allow the body to adapt and flourish as a result of that stress.

In his recent book *Antifragile: Things That Gain from Disorder*, Nassim Taleb defines the concept of antifragility as a state that not only resists, but also thrives on, uncertainty and stressors.[2] This is a perfect description for our backs—not fragile, but antifragile!

The first paradox or "hidden truth" I'll share with you involves the title of this book, *The End of Back Pain*. This book is actually *not* about the end of back pain. You will learn that back pain cannot be "ended."

Hidden Truth 1: *The End of Back Pain* Is Not the End of Back Pain!

The book will, rather, switch your focus to mitigating the back pain that will invariably rear its head. Even though back pain has no end, you will learn how to significantly reduce pain's frequency, duration, and intensity during the inevitable flare-ups.

Roth's R$_X$: Back pain is part of life. You need to learn how to maximize function and reduce pain by strengthening your back.

Focus on Philosophy
IIIIIIIIIIIIIIIIIIIIIIIIIIIIIIIIIIIIIIIIIIIIIIIIIIIIIIIIIIIIIII

The Nietzsche Principle

For many of you, this prescription will not be instinctive, but it's perhaps the most powerful of all the tools that I'll offer: Be confident in your body's remarkable ability to adapt. I call this the Nietzsche principle, named for philosopher Friedrich Nietzsche's famous utterance, "That which does not kill you makes you stronger."[3] The Nietzsche principle will be referred to throughout this book. It presents a double-edged sword that is difficult to handle: When you push yourself, you open up both the possibility of improvement and the simultaneous possibility of setback. I believe that there are times when improvement is not possible without taking this risk.

The Nietzsche principle forms the basis of my Hidden Core Workout. In other words, I will teach you how to strengthen your back—even while in pain—in order to ultimately control your pain. This is in contrast to resting your back—while in pain—in order to protect it. Working through pain isn't like banging your head against the wall with a total disregard for the pain; rather, it's a willingness to feel some pain while you slowly progress with exercise.

THE BRAIN-BODY CONNECTION

Mens sana in corpore sano is Latin for "A healthy mind in a healthy body." For the purposes of this book we should perhaps modify this to *Mens sana in spina sana,* or "A healthy mind in a healthy spine."

The brain and the spine are intertwined—not only developmentally, but functionally. One of the themes of this book is that we can leverage this relationship by applying a biological "bait-and-switch." If we rewire the brain with regard to the spine, for instance, the spine will follow suit and change. Likewise, by equipping the spine with strength, posture, and technique through exercise, we can effectively rewire the brain.

CHANGE YOUR BRAIN, CHANGE YOUR BACK AND SPINE

The brain has a crucial role in enabling health. Education has consistently been shown to be an independent enabler of health. In fact, the human brain's capacity to learn and become educated may be its most important link to health. One of the obstacles we encounter with education, however, is that some of the things we learn from our culture are outdated or even counterproductive to our health.

The term *memes,* coined by evolutionary biologist Richard Dawkins, refers to culturally relevant ideas or behaviors that are passed on from generation to generation.[4] Our brain development is profoundly affected by these cultural abstractions. As our collective view of the world becomes more sophisticated, so do the memes that are passed on to the next generation. This, in turn, allows for more sophisticated brain development in that next generation. Surprisingly, memes play an important role in pain. You will later learn that pain is significantly influenced by culturally derived expectations. In other words, your brain is developed, in part, by the culture in which it matures, and that development influences the actual pain that you feel years later when your back hurts.

> ## Core Question
> |||||||||||||||||||||||||||||||||||||||||
>
> *Can the Brain Be "Rewired" to Eliminate Pain?*
>
> There is evidence that it can. One interesting experiment, which involved patients with severe arm pain on one side, had each patient place both arms into a mirrored contraption that made the patient think that the "good" arm was the "bad" arm. When the good arm was put through range of motion, it looked to the patient as if it was the bad arm being manipulated. Since there was no pain with the range of motion (it was actually the good arm, remember), the patient was "tricked" into thinking that the bad arm was moving without pain. After several weeks of this therapy, the bad arm was no longer painful with movement.[5] This suggests that the "pain" arose in the brain and that the brain could be "rewired."

The reason I present many of the ideas in this book as "hidden truths" is to disabuse you of many of these cultural assumptions. As you shed faulty assumptions, your education can better serve to enhance, rather than diminish, your health.

In addition to education, the brain can promote health via three related essential attributes: self-efficacy (one's ability to maintain health), a willingness to take responsibility or action, and a fascinating mind-body phenomenon called embodied cognition. Let's take a look at each of those attributes in turn.

SELF-EFFICACY

Labeled by Albert Bandura, a psychologist and professor at Stanford University, self-efficacy is the capability and confidence to effect change or bring about positive results. In the promotion of your health—especially when dealing with back pain—self-efficacy is essential.[6]

How do you nurture self-efficacy? In his book *Next Medicine,* Walter Bortz, a physician who is a wellness and longevity expert, describes four key ingredients of self-efficacy:[7]

1. *Small steps:* This ingredient is emphasized in the Hidden Core Workout, where patience and slow, steady progress are paramount. In fact, I've designed the program in four stages so that you can target specific muscles at the right times for your strength level.

2. *Peer examples/role models:* This involves seeking others around you who have overcome pain and allowing the wisdom of their experience to guide you.

3. *Social persuasion:* This refers to learning the science and philosophy that pertain to your pain and becoming an active participant in the decision-making process. Just by reading this book, you're already one-quarter of your way to self-efficacy.

4. *Diminished cues of failure:* If your back hurts when you run, don't stop running. Instead, find a way to run without pain.

TAKING RESPONSIBILITY AND ACTION

Many a false step was made by standing still.
—ANONYMOUS

The brain can profoundly influence health by assuming responsibility for the promotion of health. Resolution of pain is best achieved by the individual's gaining a state of independence—independence from doctors, therapists, medications, and cultural dogmas. This state requires the brain to take action—to become an active participant by learning about the cause of the pain, when possible, and analyzing and evaluating each therapy as it's proposed and utilized.

Hidden Truth 2: Healthcare Is Not *Health* Care but *Disease* Care!

Our healthcare system spends too much time and money on treating disease. We have made fantastic progress in various disease states, such as certain infectious diseases and cancers. The time has come, however, to prioritize the promotion of health over the eradication of disease.

As a surgeon, I've been trained to understand and treat pain from a mechanical standpoint. My job is not only to interpret the relevance of a pathologic disc herniation (for example) with regard to a specific pain, but also to decide if the pain has a structural or mechanical cause. In order to root out mechanical malfunctions, I've dedicated my career to utilizing a patient's entire history—as conveyed by the patient, the physical exam, and the MRI—to determine the cause(s) of pain. No doubt I've had many successes, as there are many patients with clear structural or mechanical causes for their pain. On the other hand, I've taken credit for many successes that could more accurately be attributed to the human body's capacity to heal itself.

Voltaire once said, "The art of medicine consists in amusing the patient while nature cures the disease." Obviously, as a surgeon, I don't fully subscribe to such an impotent philosophy, but I do believe strongly in the power of nature and thus in the power of each patient.

Roth's R$_X$: Every back pain sufferer can become an active participant in facilitating the body's natural healing and shielding ability and mitigate back pain for good. To do so, put your energy into changing your body and not into seeking either a specific cause or a quick solution.

Focus on Philosophy
||||||||||||||||||||||||||||||||||||||||||||||||||||||||

The Kierkegaard Principle

You need to start your back pain treatment even before you can be sure that you're starting in the correct place. If you're provided choices, you will likely start with the more conservative treatment option. That's fine. What is essential is that you start *somewhere*. Once started, pay close attention to how you feel and the progress you make, and you can then modify and adapt your treatment plan accordingly.

This need to commit is often thwarted by an underlying fear that you don't have enough of a knowledge base to make such a decision; thus you have to take the "leap of faith" described by Danish philosopher Søren Kierkegaard.[8] Kierkegaard suggested that the "leap" could be made only when one understands that the desired knowledge base is truly unattainable. And that's certainly the case in regard to back health: You can never know enough to make a "guaranteed" correct choice. Give up this desire for empirical evidence or a crystal ball, and just leap! Perhaps Nike states the Kierkegaard principle better than Kierkegaard himself. "Just do it," the Nike ads proclaim—or, as FDR said, "Try something. If it works, do more of it. If it doesn't, do something else."

The inherent advantage to being active as a way of life, to living by the Kierkegaard principle, has resonated with me ever since learning of the arm pain experiment described earlier—the one in which test subjects moved their bad arm without pain, thinking it was the good arm. Now activity permeates my philosophy of the treatment of back pain.

EMBODIED COGNITION

The third and final form of control that the brain can exert on the body (and the body can exert on the brain) is known as embodied cognition. While responsibility creates action, embodied cognition *sustains* that action. Although philosophers and psychologists have long considered the relationship between the mind and the body to be unidirectional (the mind decides on an action and the body follows orders), embodied cognition suggests that the relationship is bidirectional. Embodied cognition is the emerging understanding that the way we think is inextricably tied to the state of our body. Or, to put it in other words, the human mind is determined by the form of the body.

Embodied cognition says that there's an inseparable link between cognition and the body itself. What we think influences how we act, and how we act influences what we think. Once we decide to take the leap of faith to action, the state of our physical body can rewire our brain. The connection between brain and body is synergistic. The mind, rather than residing solely in the brain, is embodied outside of the brain.

This concept is critical to anyone trying to build the confidence to adopt a new lifestyle—in this case, to adopt the Hidden Core Workout. Pushing your body, even when it's uncomfortable, can actually cause your mind to believe that you're something other than—and more capable than—a victim of pain. People with hip pain, for instance, have been shown to have less gray matter in their brains. After these people undergo hip surgery, and their pain has improved, their brains are found to have restored the gray matter.[9] This is a great example of a change in the body bringing about a change in the brain. It's also a great demonstration of the plasticity of the brain.

THE VIRTUAL BRAIN

The first time I used image-guided technology to remove a brain tumor, I was both awestruck and slightly tentative. We use a system that transfers the information from a magnetic resonance image (MRI) to a computer in the operating room. By touching points around the skull of the patient, the surgeon is able to get the computer to render a virtual picture of the brain; that picture can then be used to help the surgeon navigate around a tumor.

Sounds great, right? And yet, was I going to trust my eyes or this computer-generated image of the brain and the tumor? I understood that pilots flying stealth aircrafts at extreme velocities and in remote spaces don't need (and typically don't bother) to look out the window,

Core Concept

As we learn about pain throughout this book, it's important to understand that all of our "natural" perceptions are really "expert" perceptions. Here's what I mean: The brain starts with a prediction of what it will see, feel, taste, etc., and then modifies this expert prediction with an update from the involved sensory apparatus. In this regard we typically "see the forest before the trees."

In addition, our senses don't work in isolation but are integrated in and with our brain. When watching a movie, for example, we "hear" the sound coming from the actor's mouth regardless of where the speakers are actually located in the theater. In the end, then, our reality is defined by the relative contributions of our *various* sensory systems. A bloodhound, on the other hand—with its extraordinary sense of smell—constructs a very different virtual world, one that includes a disproportional amount of olfactory information.

but rather rely on computers similar to our hospital model to know where they are and where they're headed. And yet part of me wanted to rely on my "trustworthy" eyes, not this new technology, as I removed that tumor from my patient's brain.

It turns out, however, that the more we learn about the brain, the more we understand that even the "trustworthy" information that our eyes continually provide our brains as conscious experience is also "interpretive," and thus more virtual than conventional wisdom would suggest. It would require too much energy and attention to visually survey our environment *constantly,* so we spend much of our time in a virtual reality, with our eyes only intermittently updating us or interrupting us.

The brain is truly a marvel of complexity. In a three-pound package that can be held in the palm of one's hand live one hundred billion neurons, each making between one thousand and ten thousand connections. The brain is designed to read and communicate patterns that exist in nature so that complex levels of higher thinking can ultimately emerge from what starts out as a blank slate. It's also designed to adapt and flourish regardless of what environment it develops in.

Perhaps even more fascinating than the sheer complexity of the brain is the brain's capacity to create a virtual rendering of the world that it surveys. This virtual rendering goes way beyond the conscious experience of sensory stimuli. The brain constructs a virtual map of our actions, for example. This process is mediated by "mirror neurons" that not only virtually map out our movements right before they occur, but map out these movements if we merely *think* about performing a movement or if we're simply watching someone else perform a movement![10]

Similarly, the brain has a virtual pain map. Neurons in the anterior cingulate cortex, a part of the brain involved in the anticipation of pain and emotions, fires both when we have pain and when we watch someone else experiencing pain. The virtual mapping of motor activity and of pain helps explain how the social and cultural fabric that surrounds us can literally become part of us. In the next chapter you'll learn more about how the brain creates a virtual rendering of pain, which it can amplify or suppress depending on circumstances.

Remarkably, the virtual reality that the brain creates is closely linked to our body design. In other words, our brain functions in a way that reflects our ability to walk upright and to use our thumb to oppose the other fingers. In contrast, a dog's virtual reality would reflect its extraordinary sense of smell.

Human brain function became unique among animals as our neocortex, the layer that covers the brain of all mammals, expanded and developed. In humans, this covering evolved an increased surface area through folding of the surface into ridges and grooves and through the development of an enlarged frontal lobe (thus the human forehead). The human neocortex accounts for 80 percent of our three-pound brain weight.

That highly developed neocortex is responsible for what we think of as "thinking." It's responsible for our sensory perceptions, language, reasoning, planning, worrying, and movements. It also presides over our "older brain," the part of the brain that creates memories, responds to fear, regulates sleep, emotes, and regulates pain. The neocortex's interpretive relation to our "older brain" further distinguishes us from other animals.

Much has been written of the brain's so-called executive function. This refers to the ability of the neocortex (primarily the area called the prefrontal cortex) to manage and control the various cognitive functions of the brain. In this book, I introduce the term "judicial function" to describe the brain's capacity to layer an interpretive context not only on perceptual impulses from our senses, but on the perception and management of our "older brain" functions—in particular, the perception and regulation of pain. The term "judicial" is offered as a contrast to the term "executive." I will leave it to someone else to define the "legislative" function of our brain!

CHANGE YOUR BODY—CHANGE YOUR BRAIN

Hidden Truth 3: Sometimes You're Happy Because You Smile!

Sometimes effect precedes cause. Sure, we smile when we're happy, but sometimes we're happy simply because we smile. Sometimes we need to act before we think.

Such a relationship exists between using our back and back pain. Simply by using our back and strengthening our back, we alter our conception of what our back can and can't do. This is an example of embodied cognition, a fundamental principle of the Hidden Core Workout.

Roth's R$_X$: You want to be happy? Try smiling. You
want to improve your back pain? Try the old bait-and-
switch: Exercise your back correctly *without* pain and
have less pain when you use your back later.

We've seen how changing your brain can change your body. Now let's see how changing your body can change your brain—that is, how smiling can make you happy. Our first step in understanding that process is to grasp our capacity to change.

Focus on Philosophy
||||||||||||||||||||||||||||||||||||||||||||||||||||||

The Maugham Principle

Somerset Maugham suggested in his book *Of Human Bondage* that the real strength in an individual lies not in his or her ability to persist or never give up, but rather in his or her ability to change and try something new. I refer to this as the Maugham principle. The Hidden Core Workout is your chance to find out just how true this is.

THE ADAPTABLE BODY

The evolution of our species has been powered and guided by a survival advantage. Our unique adaptation for survival lies in the development of a brain that can plan, worry, and abstract. Perhaps the most important part of our genome is, however, its capacity to allow for adaptation to our environment.

Most of you are well versed in the principles of evolution and its power to be selective for, or favor, a genetic makeup that confers a survival advantage, but the related concept of epigenetics may be less familiar to you.

Epigenetics refers to that aspect of the heritable genetic makeup that allows for individual *cells* (and thus, ultimately, individuals) to adapt to stressors. Our genome allows for the formation and replication of the cell, but—perhaps more importantly—it also codes for a cell membrane that can react to its environmental stressors by turning on specific genes that can produce the necessary adaptive proteins.

Through this feature, called phenotypic plasticity, our cells are blessed with the ability to adapt to a changing environment. It couldn't be any other way, of course, as no genetic map could anticipate all the requirements of a cell living in an unpredictable environment.

An individual also has the capacity to adapt. Although this adaptation ultimately takes place on a cellular level, the cells are interdependent, as are the various organs that are composed of these cells. The adaptation of an individual thus involves an efficient distribution of adaptation in *all* the interdependent cells and organs. This distribution of adaptation is referred to as symmorphosis.[11]

A good example of symmorphosis is the reaction of the human body to exercise. The stress of exercise channels energy to individual cells throughout the body. These cells react to the stress; but, in addition, the organism as a whole reacts to the stress, and this results in a co-dependent and functionally distributed adaptation of the cardiovascular system, the muscular system, the skeletal system, and so on. Aerobic exercise may functionally affect the cardiovascular system predominantly, while weight training distributes the energy more heavily into adaptation of the muscles and skeleton, but both instances involve systemic adaptation.

Exercising stimulates the brain to produce more neurons through a process known as neurogenesis.[12] Just a few years ago, it was widely believed that neurons had no capacity to regenerate. We now know that this is not the case. The brain possesses far more plasticity than we had imagined. Scientists comparing rats that ran in their cages to those that were sedentary found a dramatic increase in stem cells (new cells that have the potential to assume many different roles) in the active group—in fact, the active rats had twice as many stem cells in the portion of their brain known as the hippocampus. This is great evidence of exercise's capacity to cause brain growth.

In addition to neuron growth, exercise causes neurons to sprout dendrites. These are the branches of the neurons that allow for networking and communication among neurons. Exercising releases a variety of factors (or proteins) that stimulate neurons. The most well known such factor is brain-derived neurotrophic factor (BDNF). In addition to bringing about dendritic sprouting, BDNF also causes proteins to be produced that facilitate nerve conduction at the synapses. Finally, exercise results in factors that help with neuron metabolism and blood supply—for example, insulin-like growth factor (IGF-1) and vascular endothelial growth factor (VEGF).

Exercise also results in an increase of serotonin, an important hormone involved in regulating anxiety and mood. That uptick in serotonin means that working the back and the body minimizes the distraction of pain and thus helps the back pain sufferer focus on the task at hand.

Exercising the back with proper form and minimal pain allows for the initiation of a biological bait-and-switch. In a person who uses the back in a controlled and successive manner, the brain learns to substitute an expectation of success for an expectation of pain.

The relation of the back to the brain is synergistic. Exercising the back and body potentiates the brain's capacity to learn; likewise, the brain's capacity to learn can potentiate health.

The Gist

- The brain and the body have a remarkable relationship. They codeveloped as we evolved, and they remain inextricably intertwined.

- The brain and the spine are each blessed with the capacity to adapt. Working on either the brain or the spine has reciprocal and synergistic effects.

- Building back health reduces pain, but it requires changing *both* our back *and* our mind.

- Education is an independent enabler of health.

- The brain can promote health through self-efficacy, responsibility and action, and embodied cognition.

CHAPTER 2

PAIN

Y OU NOW HAVE a sense of how the brain and body are intertwined. Nowhere is that interaction more evident than in the experience of pain. Instead of thinking of pain as simply the perception of a painful stimulus, you will learn, in the pages of this chapter, that pain is far more complicated.

Pain can usefully be conceptualized as having three-tiered causation:

- The painful stimulus
- The epiphenomenon (or multiple epiphenomena)
- The "judicial function" of the brain

Pain can be caused by any of these components, separately or in combination. Let's take a look at each component individually.

THE PAINFUL STIMULUS

Often back pain is simply the result of a painful stimulus. This is the most basic cause of pain, and the one that makes the most sense. Something is pushing on, or irritating, a nerve. This component of pain can easily be substantiated by our understanding of physiology and can often be demonstrated by an MRI, which may show the actual nerve being compressed.

A painful stimulus may be accentuated in two common ways. First, there may be a coexistent inflammation. Inflammation is a chemically mediated condition that can markedly amplify pain (inflammatory cells release chemicals that can result in local pain). This phenomenon is well known to any surgeon who has operated on a painful nerve root using only local anesthesia. A noninflamed nerve root doesn't cause pain when it's manipulated, while an inflamed nerve root is excruciatingly sensitive when handled. In this regard, the pain, though obviously more intense, is not unlike that caused by a splinter in the foot. Once infected, the skin around the splinter becomes ten times more painful to the touch than it was with the splinter alone.

Motion also exacerbates pain, regardless of the actual cause of pain, which is why we tend to want to rest when we're in pain. In diseases of the spine, the term *instability* is often used to describe motion of the spine. Even the smallest motion can bring about pain if there's a stimulus present.

THE EPIPHENOMENON (OR EPIPHENOMENA)

If not a result of a specific stimulus, back pain is often the result of the body's *reaction* to a painful stimulus. I call such a reaction an "epiphenomenon." Although the body's intent is to make the pain better, its reaction to a painful stimulus can, itself, paradoxically be a *source* of pain. With back pain, the three most common epiphenomena are (1) soft-tissue pain related to rest or disuse, (2) muscle spasm, and (3) postural change.

When healthy men who had no back pain were asked to go on bed for a research study, they developed back pain after a brief time similar to the pain that accompanies an injury to the back.[1] This is an example of an epiphenomenon—resting itself caused pain. I had a patient, Ron, who decided to stop exercising after performing some core exercises I'd given him for his back pain, because they hurt when he first tried them. Ironically, the resting itself became the cause of the pain after a while. Breaking Ron free from this cycle of disuse, and encouraging and teaching him how to be active, ended up helping him with his pain.

Pain often triggers the epiphenomenon of muscle spasm, the sustained, involuntary, and painful clenching of a muscle. Similarly, pain can result in the disruption of normal posture, and the subsequent persistence of that abnormal posture—even after the original painful stimulus has abated—can itself be painful. Try walking around like Groucho Marx for fifteen minutes—I guarantee you that your back will hurt.

Persistence of soft-tissue pain, muscle spasm, or postural change can have a "kindling effect"—in other words, once initiated, an epiphenomenon can grow until it ultimately establishes a nervous system "circuit" that's self-perpetuating.

THE JUDICIAL FUNCTION OF THE BRAIN

The brain is not only a passive recipient of pain, but often also an active creator of it. In addition to any given pain stimulus, the brain also has to consider and interpret a variety of other factors, such as preconceived notions, previous experience, cultural norms, and underlying anxiety. Thus pain cannot always be thought of as a direct, or mirrored, representation of the painful stimulus in the brain. In this interpretive context, the brain can *create* pain. I refer to this interpretive function as the brain's "judicial function."

ple examples of how this judicial function works.
crease or decrease the strength of the signal com-
stimulus (more on this later) before that signal
the brain. Second, the brain not only defines pain based
previous experience and culturally derived expectations, but is
wired to couple its interpretation of a stimulus with an action. This
action can range from withdrawal of one's hand from a hot object to a
much more complex behavior.

Picture a father taking his son into a hot tub for the first time. As they
step into the tub, both are confronted with hot water of the same temperature. The father has been in many hot tubs and expects the tub to
feel quite hot; more importantly, he knows that if he waits a few seconds
to acclimate, the heat will become pleasurable. The son, on the other
hand, feels the same heat but has never been in this situation. The
ultimate interpretation of the pain for each of them is tied to formulat-
ing an appropriate action. Despite the fact that the temperature is the
same for both of them, the father stands patiently while the son jumps
out. In the same setting, the son experiences more fear, and thus more
pain, than the father—despite an identical stimulus to each. You can
see that the ultimate pain is less a function of the temperature of the
water than the state of the brain.

Hidden Truth 4: Back Pain Is Not in Your Back—It's in Your Head!

Even when a heavy weight drops on your foot, the pain that's produced is "in your head." As the weight strikes your foot, pain-sensing
structures, called nociceptors, are triggered—but this is not yet pain.
It's kind of like the age-old philosophical question: "If a tree falls in the
forest and no one is around to hear it, does it make a sound?" In the
case of a tree falling, sound waves are certainly formed, but they aren't
an actual "sound" until they affect someone's auditory apparatus,

which sends its information to the brain for interpretation. The catch here is "interpretation," which (depending on the individual hearer) is subject to preconceived notions, editorializing, and previous experiences of a tree falling in the forest.

Similarly, with a painful stimulus, a sensation is not pain until the stimulus has been "processed" in the brain. In other words, pain is not pain simply because a receptor on the skin is stimulated; the pain message then has to travel to the brain, where its final representation is rendered. Going back to the sound analogy, if you were at a shooting range, the bang of a gunshot would sound drastically different than if you were alone in the forest and heard the same gun go off. It's the same sound waves in each case—but a different "sound" because of the different way your brain handles, a.k.a. "interprets," the sound waves.

Several recent studies evaluated patients with back pain and patients without back pain. The patients were examined through functional MRIs, a type of imaging that reveals areas of the brain that are active at the time of the MRI. These studies show several anatomical and functional differences between subjects with and without pain. These differences show that the brain is different in subjects with pain. It is not hard to further imagine that these differences help to substantiate the brain's role as an active creator of pain.[2] Successful treatment of the pain with a variety of different methods, such as physical therapy, can reverse or rectify some of these anatomical brain changes, further indicating the brain's role in some instances of pain.

Not surprisingly (given the brain-body connection), both cognitive therapy and exercise have been shown to be as effective as fusion surgery in the treatment of back pain. The efficacy of these therapies likely stems from their effect on any epiphenomenal and judicial function aspects of pain, and not on the original painful stimulus. These non-surgical treatments are often more cost-effective and require less time out of work than surgery.

Focus on Philosophy
||||||||||||||||||||||||||||||||||||||||||||||||||||||||||

René Descartes

The conceptualization of pain has a long and rich history. I always find it useful to begin with an old-fashioned theory popularized by, and partially credited to, the philosopher René Descartes. This theory suggests that with pain there are always two separate entities: the painful stimulus and the perception or representation of that stimulus in the brain. The stimulus and its representation are distinct and should be thought of separately. To Descartes's mind, there was the "real" world and there was the distinct representation of that world in the brain.

This dualistic conception of pain was found to have serious flaws, however—as you will see—and there has evolved a more "modern" theory of pain. The modern theory looks at pain as an active output from the brain rather than the brain's passive rendering of an input from the outside. This paradigm shift occurred in reaction to two findings that made the old theory untenable. First, pain can arise from or be triggered by factors unrelated to physical harm or tissue injury (as noted earlier). This phenomenon is the basis of chronic pain and will be explored in greater detail later in the chapter. Second, in other circumstances, pain can be conspicuously absent even when there's a significant and obvious ongoing painful stimulus. For example, soldiers have had their limbs blown off in battle and yet have felt no pain for hours as they made their way to safety.[3]

Pain, then, is a complex integration of a stimulus (a heavy weight, for example), the expectation of that stimulus (a weight is supposed to be heavy), and a learned response to that stimulus (a bruise throbs for days). The brain's role in interpreting a stimulus and determining an appropriate level of pain is known as its judicial function. Essentially, the brain acts like a judge, weighing the various elements to decide if there is pain and, if so, to what degree.

Moreover, that "interpretation" and "molding" of the stimulus by the brain is done with a purpose: to form a reaction to the pain (for example, pull the foot away). In other words, the ultimate interpretation of the brain to a stimulus is closely coupled with a need to act—likely a trait tied to survival.

HOW PAIN FINDS ITS WAY TO THE BRAIN

The human nervous system is divided into two connected systems: the central nervous system, which includes the brain and the spinal cord, and the peripheral nervous system. The peripheral nervous system is made up of motor nerves, which travel from the brain to the muscles, and sensory nerves, which transmit information gathered through the senses back to the brain. Both types of nerves are covered by a conductive material called myelin, which enables quick transmission of information.

A subgroup of sensory nerves uses small nerve fibers to transmit information to the brain regarding pain and temperature, but in a slower manner. If you touch a hot object, for example, you will "feel" it before you consciously know that it's hot; this is due to the relatively quicker transmission of the larger sensory nerves. The slightly delayed "brain freeze" that's apparent a second after eating cold ice cream is an example of the slower transmission.

Pain nerves never connect directly to the brain; rather, they "synapse," or form connections with, a second group of nerves that *do* connect to the brain. This extra step gives the brain an opportunity to influence what it experiences in terms of pain. The brain can either facilitate this connection and increase pain, or inhibit this connection and diminish pain. The brain exerts this control by sending its own impulses down to the synapses, those links where the first sensory nerve connects to the second (brain-contacting) sensory nerve. The impulse from the brain can alter the environment in the synapse in such a way as to either inhibit or facilitate the passing on of the transmission that originated from the painful stimulus. This is why I said earlier that the representation of pain in the brain is fundamentally different from the stimulus: The brain sets its own threshold for pain to get through, depending on how important the brain views the pain. An example of the brain using its descending control in diminishing pain may be the learned ability of some people to walk on hot coals without apparent pain.

THE GATE CONTROL THEORY OF PAIN

The synapses that separate the brain from the pain nerves that receive the initial painful stimulation are influenced not only by the brain, as we just saw, but also by the faster and parallel-running sensory nerves of vibration and touch for the same area of the body. In other words, when a painful stimulus triggers a sensory nerve to "fire," that transmission has to go through a connection before getting to the brain— and that connection is regulated not only by the brain (with the fibers that it sends down to the synapse), but also by the nerves that supply the sensation of touch. This dual regulation is a pain inhibitor, according to the so-called gate control theory of pain.

   This theory says that in a painful event, if there's simultaneous sensation from the same part of the body that's experiencing pain, then this simultaneous sensation can inhibit the transmission of the painful stimulant and thus result in less pain. An example of using this to your advantage is gently pressing on your head when you have a headache, to help diminish the pain. The idea is to flood the central nervous system with additional sensation (the pressure applied to the temple), therefore inhibiting the synapses of the pain transmission.

As a neurosurgeon, I've occasionally used a tool called a dorsal column stimulator, which is thought to work via the gate control theory of pain. This device, placed into the spine over the spinal cord, causes stimulation of the large sensory fibers and, in turn, diminishes the pain. The patient feels only a "buzzing" or vibration in the area that was formerly painful. This new sensation is generally preferable to the patient. Once implanted, the dorsal column stimulator can be fine-tuned by a magnet.

Ultimately, the pain transmission is received in an area of the brain called the thalamus. From the thalamus there are further connections to the limbic system (which governs emotions), the motor strip (which governs muscle movement), and other parts of the cerebral cortex. Via these final connections, pain, having been received by the brain, is automatically adjusted by the emotional part of the brain and then sent to the motor part of the brain for response. These connections substantiate the modern theory of pain by providing evidence that any given stimulus is anatomically linked to those parts of the brain that can interpret and act.

THE PLACEBO EFFECT

Now that you have an overview of how the brain can and does alter pain, it's time to look at the placebo effect, along with something you've likely never heard of, the nocebo effect. Rather than thinking of these concepts as illusory or pseudoscientific, consider the paradoxical possibility that the virtual capability of our brain (as discussed in chapter 1) is the true purveyor of pain and that the "scientific" basis of, for example, pain medication should be demoted to the status of "merely tapping into the placebo effect"!

John Sarno
||||||||||||||||||||||||||||

The Guy Who Says It's All in Your Head

Dr. John Sarno remains a top-selling author more than twenty years after the publication of his popular book *Healing Back Pain: The Mind-Body Connection.* Although he's had widespread criticism from parts of the medical community, Sarno provides statistical and anecdotal evidence to support his success in treating back pain. In the office, I'm often asked whether reading the book "by the guy who says that it's all in your head" would be valuable. I always encourage my patients to read Sarno's book and give his approach a try; however, I don't fully agree with the book's philosophy and reasoning.

Sarno states that pain is a physical (somatic) manifestation of an underlying anxiety, fear, or rage. He sees pain as a "brain-mediated" restriction of oxygen to the muscles (with resultant pain from the lack of oxygen). Sarno claims further that pain arises from a muscular syndrome that he calls tension myositis syndrome. He believes that the syndrome is psychosomatic—the body creating a physical distraction to divert attention from painful underlying psychological issues. The theory is provocative and compelling, but the component of pain being generated from lack of oxygen (hypoxia) to muscles has little scientific backing.

It's important to point out that Sarno does *not* suggest that pain isn't real; rather, he posits that traditional treatments will likely be a waste of time in easing pain. The pain should be treated, he states, by recognizing the origin of the pain as a somatic manifestation of repressed emotions. Once this acknowledgment takes place, the pain often recedes. As the pain recedes, the patient is instructed to resume his or her typical activities.

Sarno's remarkable reported successes lend credibility to his theory, but, as stated above, I believe that his speculated hypoxia to muscles is unlikely to be the actual cause of the pain. I would suggest, alternatively, that the perception of pain is simply a complicated behavioral response to a stimulus that persists because the brain believes that a *new* pain that's been created in response to a different stimulus is "less painful" than the preexisting pain that it has displaced.

A classic example of this would be the young manual laborer who develops a sore back at work. Prior to that episode, he had been fighting with his wife and was under the impression that she was ready to leave him. With the new back pain, the fighting at home is put on hold and the wife tries to help her hurting husband. While this is going on, the brain of the laborer is focused on diminishing pain. Again, this is a natural trait of the brain. In this setting, however, the brain is forced to weigh and compare two pains: the back pain and the pain of his relationship. For the laborer, the back pain displaces the relationship pain, and the brain looks at this displacement as providing less pain overall. It, in turn, utilizes its active role to "facilitate" the back pain and thus lower *overall* pain. Basically, the laborer allows himself to feel increased chronic back pain to avoid his relationship problems.

Understanding the placebo effect is critical to understanding pain. The term *placebo* is derived from the Latin "I shall please," and it originally had a church connection as part of the vespers service for the dead. Its shady reputation stems back hundreds of years to a time when the term was applied to priests who were paid to mourn at funerals.

Placebo use has a rich history in medicine as well. The placebo effect is defined loosely as an effect that occurs simply because it's *expected* to occur. I argue that the placebo effect is widely used in a nondeliberate sense today[4]—that is, doctors prescribe medicines or treatments in the *hope* that those medicines will improve symptoms, and they in fact do help, but only because they're *expected* to—and that sort of usage goes back centuries. When a medicine or treatment that's *known* to be useless is nonetheless prescribed—that is, when the placebo effect is *deliberately* applied—it has a quality of deceit (as with the paid mourners) that taints its application.

The old practice of bloodletting is an example of the nondeliberate use of a placebo. Suppose a patient presented a thousand years ago with chronic abdominal pain. His physician likely conducted bloodletting to allow the "evil humors" to escape. Following the procedure, the patient's abdominal pain may indeed have resolved. We now know that any improvement had nothing to do with the treatment itself, but what *did* allow for improvement? Most likely, in part, the placebo effect. That's true of many of the treatments in medicine that were subsequently abandoned as a better understanding of the disease in question brought on newer, better treatments. It can be argued that the "successes" of those previous, abandoned treatments—which were in fact sometimes followed by improved health—were, in part, mediated by the placebo effect. When we look back at some of those ancient treatments we tend to cringe, and yet enough patients were seen to improve to "validate" those treatments.

What separates such treatments philosophically from an *engineered* placebo treatment today is only the intent. Though many of the treatments in the past had no rationale in retrospect, they were delivered earnestly. That doesn't mean, however, that their effectiveness wasn't related to the placebo effect. In 1860, Oliver Wendell Holmes suggested that "it would be better for mankind if all the drugs of the day could be sunk to the bottom of the sea—and all the worse for the fishes." In retrospect, he was correct in terms of rationale, but not necessarily in terms of effect.

There's one other factor that helps explain the success of past medical practices that have subsequently been discovered to be shams, and that's something called "regression to the mean." This is the idea that when we experience a symptom that's unusual, it's likely to go away simply because we don't "usually" experience that symptom. In other words, some conditions just get better on their own. This phenomenon has recently been looked at as playing an overlooked part in the improvement of patients that seem to respond to a placebo. In fact, when any treatment is compared to a placebo, the study should also include a "no treatment" group to separate out the possibility of regression to the mean.

Although the placebo effect has been around as long as doctors have been treating patients, it began to gain serious attention after a study looking at treatment of chest pain was conducted more than fifty years ago by Leonard Cobb. In that study, the procedure of tying off the internal mammary artery was compared with a sham operation in which the skin was cut, but the artery was not tied off. The study showed that both groups had less subsequent chest pain.[5]

PLACEBOS AND PAIN

How do placebos work? Clearly, it's not purely a physical phenomenon, because when placebos are given without a patient's knowledge that *any* drug is being administered, they have no effect. Just as clearly, placebos aren't purely manifested mentally. An experiment in which subjects were given decaffeinated coffee in place of the expected caffeinated coffee showed not only a sense of alertness in the patient, but also a demonstrated tremulousness that would normally be seen only with caffeine. Placebos more likely ignite the brain's own pain-stifling mechanism. This involves a combination of expectation *and* the ability of the brain to engage its inherent and learned ability to lessen the painful response to a stimulus. This conclusion is supported by functional MRI studies showing that when a subject thinks he's getting a narcotic (but isn't), the brain releases endorphins (natural pain killers), and when the subject thinks the narcotics are being stopped, the hippocampus (the memory and anxiety center) becomes active.

The fact that a placebo can ignite this system of pain modification must be seen as evidence of the brain's participation not only in the *reception* of pain, but also in the *modification* of pain and the *perpetuation* of chronic pain.

THE NOCEBO EFFECT

Just as there's an endogenous pain regulation system that can be "tapped into" by simply expecting a pain to improve (the placebo effect), a similar regulatory system exists—and can be "tapped into"— that results in the creation or exacerbation of pain.

There is, in fact, the "nocebo effect," from the Latin "I will harm," which reflects the power of negative thinking. I view the syndrome of chronic pain as a manifestation of the nocebo effect. You will see later that chronic pain isn't simply pain that's present for a long time; rather, it's pain that persists despite no apparent stimulus. This happens because, just as the brain's judicial function can stifle pain via the placebo effect, it can create or amplify pain via the nocebo effect.

When we take pain medication, we're really merely tapping into a broader placebo effect; the meds are simply binding to receptors that our natural endorphins utilize. In fact, then, making a distinction between "real" treatment and placebo treatment is misleading. Similarly, all pain—even something as mundane as stubbing one's toe—can be conceptualized as merely the result of tapping into the nocebo effect.

The history of narcotics involves the fortuitous discovery of various natural substances that just happen to bind to the receptors that the body uses to control pain naturally. Taking pain medication to control pain is no more "real" than any other method we use to tap into our natural pain control system. The placebo effect is the facilitation or initiation of our own natural system of pain control, and pain medication is merely one of many ways of getting this done!

You now have a basic definition of pain, the understanding that pain is, at times, separate and distinct from any pain-generating stimulus, and the link of pain to an action aimed at relieving the pain. Now think back to our discussion of the virtual brain in chapter 1: Just as even our trusted sense of vision has a prominent virtual component, our pain can be conceptualized as a virtual reality. The causes and medical treatments of pain, including use of the placebo effect, should be conceptually demoted to the status of merely igniting a virtual machine that is always idling.

THE PURPOSE AND PRIORITY OF PAIN

Pain is the most common reason that people seek medical help in the United States. Pain is widespread because experiencing it is built into our DNA. Although often unpleasant, pain serves to protect us and keep us alive. A condition called congenital analgesia was recently spotlighted by the character Ronald Niedermann in Stieg Larsson's book *The Girl with the Dragon Tattoo*. Niedermann uses his insensitivity to pain to his advantage during physical altercations. To any pain sufferer, this might seem like a good condition to have, and yet these patients typically die young as a result of complications of not feeling pain. It's a reminder that pain serves a protective role in our lives, that though pain can be annoying, it's a necessity.

While people like Ronald Niedermann feel no pain, many of us feel too much. Out of all the sensations we feel in a day, how does our brain decide what is *pain* and thus is worth paying immediate attention to?

I find it helpful to start off with the concept of multitasking. Although there are some people out there who believe that they can multitask, the truth is that while our brain can take on two cognitive tasks at the same time, each will be diminished in how well we perform it. If the second task is an "easy" task that's been performed many times in the past, it can be done simultaneously with a more complicated task. An example is our ability to eat and carry on a complicated conversation at the same time, or drive to work while listening to a book on tape in the car. In the latter case, when we reach our destination we may have no memory of making all the necessary turns to get to work (indicating that our attention was elsewhere).

This relative inability to multitask can be explained by the brain's built-in filtering mechanism, which allows us to focus on a specific task. If this weren't present, all of the ambient sounds, smells, and other potential distractions would interfere with the task at hand. Instead, we possess the ability to focus on the important item and cut out extraneous "noise." When we're interrupted by pain, the pain *demands* that we stop whatever we're doing to deal with it. This is an evolved and necessary trait that competes with our ability to focus and stay on task. How, then, does the brain prioritize these two competing traits? The answer isn't fully known, but the issue is a crucial one: One of the answers to the treatment of pain may lie in a disturbance of the competition between needing to be interrupted and needing to stay on task.

Science has revealed that pain's ability to interrupt our focus is dependent on several aspects of that pain. First is the *intensity* of pain. It makes perfect sense that a stronger pain is more likely to get our attention. The second important attribute of pain is its *novelty*. If we have chronic pain in the foot, for example, and that becomes more intense, it may not necessarily grab our attention. If there's a new pain in the other foot, however, this may be deemed much more worthy of our attention. A third aspect of pain that amplifies its relative importance is its *perceived threat*. The perceived threat of pain is interesting because not only does it lead to a higher likelihood of interruption of our attention, but it also plays a part in the brain's active role of "editorializing" and, ultimately, "producing" the pain rather than simply causing us to feel it.

The idea that the mere perceived threat of pain can influence our ability to focus should therefore not be a surprise. What may be surprising, however, is that in addition to these above-described elements of the pain itself, the ability of pain to disrupt our consciousness is related to our emotional or psychological state at the time of the pain. In other words, if we're psychologically "primed" (that is, in a vulnerable state), pain can more easily interrupt us. What makes this so interesting to me is that it allows for potential intervention.

These "primed" or vulnerable states are the subject of ongoing research. One of the several states that have been identified is that of being "somatic"—that is, having a heightened level of awareness of bodily sensations. If, for instance, you're given the diagnosis of cancer, you may begin to interpret every sensation you feel as a potential spread of the cancer. Soon, you're not only reacting negatively to what you feel, but you're *looking* for sensations out of fear. With chronic back pain this seems to be common. People without chronic back pain don't panic when they feel a pain in their back, but those with chronic back pain do. This is because the "cause" of the chronic back pain—unlike the acute pain one gets when stepping on a nail, for example—is often unknown. Where there's little information, anxiety increases; and where there's increased anxiety, the pain increases; and the pain cycle ensues. This can easily transform into a somatic state (where *all* sensations are scrutinized).

Another "primed" state is pessimism—the tendency to assume a bad outcome or to exaggerate events, the proverbial glass-half-empty personality. A pessimistic person is more likely to allow a particular pain to interrupt his or her ability to focus. Such a person may also experience an exaggerated version of the "same" pain that might otherwise be well tolerated by another person.[6]

If we're psychologically "primed" to allow pain to interrupt us, wouldn't it be logical to think that this allows for potential intervention?

Hidden Truth 5: "Let Pain Be Your Guide" Is Dangerous Advice!

Here's the fifth paradox: The common, well-intentioned, and practical-seeming tenet "Let pain be your guide," if applied when you're attempting to restore function, is misguided and can paradoxically *cause* pain! In fact, this innocent assertion often results in back pain because it's used to justify passivity. (Even the road to *back*-hell is paved with good intentions!) A more appropriate tenet would be "Tolerate the pain and methodically regain function; then take the opportunity to change your back so that the problem is less likely to happen again."

When I see patients, I forewarn them with this thought: The initial action that you deploy may at first serve to increase your pain, which may cause you to think that you've made the wrong choice and need to change your approach. Don't assume that all pain is a warning. Be patient and persistent.

My patient Ron, whom I introduced earlier in the chapter, came to my office with a history of recurrent exacerbations of back pain. In between episodes, he had little in the way of pain. It seemed to him, however, that the frequency of these exacerbations was increasing and that the simplest tasks were now triggering the pain. I explained to him that proper strengthening of his core would likely make the frequency decrease. Giving him several exercises to do, I asked him to come back in a month for a follow-up appointment.

When I saw him again, he reported that the day after his first visit he tried the exercises, which brought on another exacerbation. Three days later he was better, but unwilling to continue the exercises for fear he would hurt himself. He then did nothing for twenty-seven more days until his follow-up appointment with me! Our appointment was spent with me assuring Ron that these setbacks were part of the process and that he should have returned to the routine as soon as he felt better. I explained that it might take a few exercise sessions to actually make progress. Fortified by this reassurance, he went home and resumed the exercise regimen. He returned to my office two months later feeling stronger and more confident. During long-term follow-up he has reported far less frequent exacerbations.

Ron subscribed to one of the greatest misconceptions about reacting to and treating pain: When you feel pain, tension . . . rest.

How do we move forward from this myth? The Hidden Core Workout is an active and aggressive answer to the treatment of back pain that includes the philosophies of abolishing outdated ideas of treating pain (such as this one) and embracing a nonsedentary lifestyle in an effort to improve one's back. I urge you to have patience in the period of restoring function, because sometimes, in cases like Ron's, taking this active approach results in a temporary setback.

Roth's R$_X$: Don't assume that pain is a warning to abandon your program of exercise. Experiencing pain is common and, at times, necessary. In those rare cases where the pain is progressive or is persistently present, *then* it may be necessary to let pain be your guide.

THE CRITICAL DISTINCTION
BETWEEN PAIN AND DISABILITY

In order to understand back pain, as well as the science and treatment of pain in general, it's helpful to understand that there's a distinction between back pain and disability from back pain, even though culturally we don't see those concepts as different.[7]

Anywhere in this world, from the United States to Africa, rural to urban areas, wealthy suburbs to poverty-stricken towns, there's a high prevalence of back pain. If you were to conduct a survey in all these various areas to measure who has, or recently has had, back pain, the results would be the same. In fact, nearly four out of every five people will be afflicted by back pain at some time in their life![8]

More surprising, however, is that if you were to go to these same disparate areas and conduct a survey of the prevalence of *disability* from back pain as opposed to back pain itself, the numbers would vary dramatically. To a large extent, back pain disability is a phenomenon of Westernized societies. Some non-Westernized societies don't even have a word in their language that conveys the concept of disability from back pain. In these societies, back pain is conceived, rather, as something that comes and goes like a common cold, and is merely a typical, albeit annoying, recurring part of life.

The disparity in the prevalence of disability from back pain may be the result of differing legal systems or reimbursement patterns that reward those with back pain. For the purposes of this book, however, what's relevant isn't seeing specific differences in various cultures in terms of their indemnification of back pain, but simply recognizing that when a price is put on a symptom, it may be transformed into a disease. Westernized societies have different laws and cultural biases, to be sure, and these differences have created a separation between the reality of back pain and the idea of disability due to back pain. Because our perceptions are formed by language use and customs in terms of disability and pain, we can't help but form varying ideas about how to treat that pain or react to it. To recognize this linkage brings power, because we can take control of how we choose to perceive pain and form a new plan to minimize it.[9]

HOW BACK PAIN BECAME A DISEASE

Many examples of pain may be more properly thought of as the ups and downs of life than as manifestations of an injury or "something broken."

For instance, when we get a headache, most of us accept it (though we may whine about it also), and we usually expect it to pass as mysteriously as it arose. Maybe we had a long day at work, stared at a computer screen too long, didn't get a full night's sleep, or spent the morning with cranky children. Whatever the case, we write off the headache as a reaction to something, and move on with the rest of our day.

However, what if a new MRI study were to come out showing that headaches were visible as a change in signal on the surface of the brain? Several things might be expected to occur: First, a headache would be looked at as an "injury" rather than a symptom. Second, the "injury" would become indemnified (worth money). Third, and most importantly, the actual incidence of headaches would subsequently increase! This ties back to both the chameleon effect and the concept of linguistic determinism. It's not that the headaches would be any different; it's just that each headache would no longer be a symptom, but a disease. Furthermore, knowing that an MRI had showed "something wrong" might result in anxiety and more intense headaches.

Finally, many "treatments" would arise for headaches. When a headache vanished (as it often does on its own), whatever treatment was used would be given credit for alleviating the headache. This process would become expensive and ingrained into our cultural mindset. The natural ebb and flow of headaches would be forgotten. That is in fact what's happened with back pain.

Families and friends also propagate certain conceptions of back pain, urging, "There must be something broken," or "You can't work until your back is fixed." These prevailing attitudes are outdated and can be extremely counterproductive. This book argues for a revolution of sorts in the concept of back pain and explains that the majority of pain is not related to "something broken"; rather, it represents a common, fluctuating condition of normal life. Therefore, the appropriate treatment of this pain is to facilitate the body's natural healing and shielding ability and mitigate back pain for good.

Core Concept
||||||||||||||||||||||||||||||||||||||

In 1934 surgeons William Mixter and Joseph Barr published a landmark paper that accurately depicted the role of a herniated disc in the spine as a cause of back and leg pain. As important as this intellectual milestone was, I can't help but reference the myth of Prometheus, in which fire was stolen from the Greek gods and given to humanity. Or perhaps Pandora's Box is a better myth to cite for the purposes of this publication, which allowed for the "medicalization" of back pain by providing "evidence" for the pain. Later, the proliferation of MRI machines further exacerbated the problem, making diagnosis of a herniated disc easy and unequivocal.

This easy label of "herniated disc" is an example of linguistic determinism, a premise which holds that how we *talk* about things changes how we *think* about them. If it sounds important, dangerous, and serious, then it must be . . . right? Wrong. What *is* important, dangerous, and serious, however, is the way in which the diagnosis affects the symptoms. In the book *Sway: The Irresistible Pull of Irrational Behavior,* authors Ori and Rom Brafman provide ample evidence that shows how giving someone a diagnosis leads to that person's taking on the role that the diagnosis suggests.

A diagnosis can thus be self-fulfilling. A patient's taking on the characteristics of the given diagnosis is called the chameleon effect. Just as chameleons really can change color, people can actually change their condition based on a diagnosis.

Even though there may be no clinical difference between a disc bulge, a disc herniation, and a disc extrusion, or between compression and impingement—all labels common in the field of back pain—there may be psychological and legal differences. Since there's no "standardization" in the terminology, radiologists and other clinicians are free to use whatever terms they choose.

Medicine's obsession with diagnostic language rages on despite the fact that MRIs done on symptomless patients routinely show disc disease.[10] If you look at an MRI of the lumbar spine of any random forty-year-old, you'll see something that could potentially cause pain. In other words, in the evaluation of pain, the concept of distinguishing between true—and true and unrelated—comes up over and over again. True, the patient has pain; true, the patient has a disc herniation on MRI—but these two truths are usually unrelated. This dilemma can, in part, be attributed to our inability to accept back pain as a natural fluctuation of life and our anxiety over not knowing the cause of our pain. But also consider that this need to associate pain with a cause is a result of healthcare providers feeling pressure to provide an explanation. The answer "I don't know" is seen as a sign of weakness or ignorance. This motivates doctors to provide answers that divert, or that may not be true or helpful, in an effort to satisfy the human instinct to abate fear.

Friedrich Nietzsche wrote: "The supposed instinct for causality is only fear of the unfamiliar and the attempt to discover something familiar in it—a search, not for causes, but for the familiar."[11] In the twenty-first century, we might simply call this idea a cop-out.

A friend of mine once told me that when his young son asked him, "What is sex?" he answered, "It's your gender—whether you're male or female." Technically, the father wasn't lying, but he wasn't answering the question either. His reply was a cop-out. It was a clever way of answering the question while avoiding answering the question. Similarly, I can tell a patient that she has degenerative disc disease. That will satisfy her fear of not knowing what's wrong, and give her the much-needed "cause" she's searching for—but it doesn't answer the real question, which is, "Why do I have pain?"

In many ways back pain is like the common headache or common cold—something that comes occasionally and then goes away. Instead of accepting the nuisance of back pain as we do the headache or cold, we've been conditioned to perceive back pain as dangerous; or requiring surgery or medical attention for it to go away; or as something that should not be exercised lest it get worse. These prevailing notions are the misconceptions that have converted back pain into a disease.

Hidden Truth 6: Working Hard Is Hardly Working!

Until the mid-twentieth century, there was virtually no long-term disability from back pain; although people certainly had back pain, they chose to keep working. The last sixty years have seen a steady increase in time spent out of work despite a simultaneous reduction in the number of jobs that require heavy labor. In other words, the easier our jobs have become physically, the more likely we are to have periods that we can't work due to back pain!

Most people would assume that the general wear and tear of physical work would lead to the specific wear and tear that's seen in our discs (so clearly revealed now with MRIs). This assumption is, as you might now surmise, wrong. In fact, changes that develop in our discs with age are largely genetically determined. Furthermore, any wear and tear that results from physical work may be a *positive* influence rather than a *negative* one (a paradox that I'll explain below). Finally, pain in the back has little correlation with the appearance of a laborer's discs. It's more highly correlated to his or her job satisfaction and attitude.

A study in Finland that compared the spines of twins reached some surprising conclusions. The research revealed that any extra body weight in one twin seemed to correlate with discs that appeared younger and healthier—probably, the researchers concluded, as a result of the additional wear and tear that the extra weight inflicted.[12] The study also found that a lifestyle of more physical labor was correlated with younger-appearing discs. All of the study participants showed aging of the discs over time, but stressing the back was shown to slow down the changes by causing the discs to adapt—perhaps by increasing the percentage of proteoglycans (substances within each disc that retain to water and form the gel that the disc nucleus is comprised of).

In other words, if you discover that you have degenerative disc disease, blame your parents and not your employer! And don't assume that you're condemned to a painful future. Ironically, these wear-and-tear changes in the discs often have very little to do with pain. And even where pain is involved, don't assume that disability lies ahead. It turns out that time missed at work because of back pain has little to do with what the MRI shows and a great deal to do with attitudes that are shared by coworkers and by families and friends of workers.

Two studies looked at workers who chose to remain at work despite back pain. These studies analyzed the workers' attitude toward work. One group was in the Netherlands, in a suburban setting; the other was in a rural section of New Zealand, on a farm. In both sets of workers, findings suggested that a positive attitude toward the workplace was important. In addition, the acceptance of back pain as a common and long-term problem seemed to be helpful in coping with the daily pain.[13]

One of my patients, Brian, who came to me with a work-related back injury, was an emotional wreck on his first visit. He had been a manual laborer his entire life—he was in his midthirties—and was now unable to work because of back pain. He truly believed that there was no answer to his problem. His wife was home with his young children and he needed to support them, but how? He felt that it would be impossible to learn a new trade, given his educational background and lack of experience in any other occupation.

Brian had only wear-and-tear changes visible on his MRI and was thus clearly not a candidate for surgery. We brought about several changes that were ultimately successful. First, I helped Brian understand that his pain was not related to an injury but was, rather, a typical exacerbation of low back pain that would not preclude him from returning to his job. With this information, he lost his fear. Second, after Brian explained the situation to his employer, the man gave him the latitude to "take it easy" for very brief periods when his pain was particularly bad. This gave Brian a sense of personal control. Finally, he was assured of access back to me. Although I knew that this would not be necessary, it gave him security.

What's remarkable in this case is that what started out as a desperate situation with "no good options" transitioned to a successful return to work with little actually done other than verbally giving Brian knowledge, control, and security. This transition had nothing to do with whatever was "causing the pain."

Roth's R$_X$: Stop focusing on why work is bad for your back and focus, rather, on how *you* can find ways to cope with your pain and enjoy work. Don't think of yourself as "genetically cursed"; rather, be glad that you can control your genetics, to an extent, with exercise. Work will not "break down" your back. On the contrary, your back will adapt to that work and become stronger.

PAIN: ACUTE OR CHRONIC? WHAT'S THE DIFFERENCE?

Pain is often characterized as acute or chronic. While the two types of pain are generally defined by the duration for which they last, this distinction involves much more than time. Pain is generally considered chronic when it lasts for more than six months, but the more important distinction has to do with the active role of the brain: Chronic pain typically endures long after the painful stimulus has receded or has been repaired; in other words, with chronic pain the brain manifests pain when there's no longer a pain stimulus. Interestingly, even the language that patients use to describe acute and chronic pain differs. Acute pain if often described by terms such as "sharp" or "stabbing," while chronic pain typically involves more affective terms such as "exhausting" or "sickening."

Once the difference between acute and chronic pain is understood, it should be obvious why we, as healthcare providers, are generally poor at helping chronic pain. After all, if there's no stimulus, what are we to treat? As a result, the message that patients receive regarding their chronic pain is often, "It's in your head," which is devastating to hear. This leaves patients with a sense of alienation, which further contributes to the pain.

In addition, the path of least resistance is often to give these patients pain medication because it's a quick solution and it eliminates the educational encounters that some of these patients need. Unfortunately, it's also an ineffective solution.

Hidden Truth 7: Acute Pain Needs No Treatment
and Chronic Pain Has No Treatment!

There are, of course, exceptions to this truth, or I would be out a job. The point I want to drive home is this: *Acute* back pain has a favorable "natural history." By that I mean that if nothing is done to treat it, the back pain will usually improve on its own over a period of weeks. Throughout the different discussions in this book, you will learn that many healthcare providers have capitalized on acute back pain's favorable tendency to go away on its own, only to take credit for what would have occurred without intervention. Or, to again quote the words of Voltaire, "The art of medicine consists in amusing the patient while nature cures the disease."

Chronic back pain, however, is a different story. It has a less favorable prognosis. This is related to the brain's role in creating or maintaining chronic pain. Many healthcare providers will attempt to treat it and fall short.

Roth's R$_X$: It's essential that you understand the difference between acute and chronic back pain. Luckily, both can be improved with exercise.

THE HIDDEN CORE WORKOUT AND PAIN

Where does all this lead us? You now understand that pain is, in part, mediated by the brain. You also now know that our culture can convert the natural occurrence of pain into a disability, or the innocent symptoms of pain into a disease. I will now try to convince you that my exercise program, the Hidden Core Workout, will empower you by freeing you from the negative influence of culture. It will reduce back pain and, more importantly, reduce disability. Let's see how the program can mitigate the aforementioned three aspects of pain:

The Painful Stimulus

Obviously, core strengthening has nothing to do with a painful stimulus. If you remember, however, one of the contributing factors to painful stimulus is movement. Well, what if you could strengthen your core in such a way that you would build a virtual brace around your back, thereby reducing movement of the spine? The Hidden Core Workout does this—and the beauty of it is that it almost doesn't matter where or what the original pain stimulus was. You will see that simply by learning to immobilize your back, you will cause your pain to diminish and reduce the occurrence of future pain.

Back Pain and the Emperor's New Clothes

I have a vivid memory of being a second-year medical student and taking an early course on physical diagnosis. There were about twenty of us in a room with an esteemed cardiologist and his patient. We had just learned about the various heart sounds to listen for using a stethoscope. All of us were given the opportunity to listen to the patient's heart. Then the cardiologist solicited our individual findings.

As the other students eloquently described their findings, I awaited my turn nervously. I was terrified because I had heard nothing. I made sure to remember what another student had said because I knew he was smart, and I figured that if I echoed his findings, I wouldn't be found out.

When my turn came, though, I stated simply, "I heard nothing." When the exercise was complete, the cardiologist singled me out because I was the only one in the room who'd said he'd been unable to hear anything. I flushed until he also informed the room that the patient's heart was anomalously located on the other side of the chest, meaning it was unlikely that the others could have heard what they claimed to have heard.

This is my version of Hans Christian Andersen's story "The Emperor's New Clothes." Just like the emperor and his subjects, who wouldn't admit that they couldn't see the clothes tailored by swindlers, the students in my class chose to admit to hearing something that wasn't there, rather than risk seeming unfit for medical school. Is there a similar phenomenon in the treatment of back pain today? Since it's well established that most back pain has a relatively benign course, how do we rationalize the extraordinary volume of back pain treatment rendered in many Western countries? Much of the motivation for treatment today is the hope of real success, but part of what motivates some treatment, some of the time, is the financial reward.

The Epiphenomenon

Any secondary pain or side effect of the stimulus that arises due to inactivity, postural change, or muscle spasm is also addressed through the Hidden Core Workout. Core strengthening results in increased blood flow to the back muscles, which also heats the connective tissues.

The strengthening reduces the likelihood of muscle spasm. Core strengthening also improves posture, which can result in a better balance of the spine so that the muscles that promote balance can relax. If you're tipped forward, for example, the muscles in your back have to work overtime to keep you straight. Once balance is achieved, these muscles can relax.

The Judicial Function of the Brain

The final aspect of pain is the brain's influence on how the stimulus is interpreted. The strengthening of the Hidden Core Workout plays a role here as well! One of the ways to alter the brain's interpretation of pain is to carry out tasks that the brain may expect to be dangerous and pain-provoking. If these tasks can be performed without an increase in pain, then the brain's perception of such motions will be altered.

Do you remember that certain emotional states allow for pain to advantageously compete with the task at hand for a place in our consciousness—states such as fear, anxiety, lack of confidence, and previous failure? As a form of exercise, the Hidden Core Workout often improves anxiety and depression, which can both serve as pain amplifiers. Hidden core strengthening also diminishes the novelty of the pain and the perceived threat of the pain.

Let's move on, in the next chapter, to the anatomy of the back, and then we'll address how we strengthen our hidden core.

The Gist

- Pain can be conceptualized as being caused by a stimulus, an epiphenomenon, and/or the judicial function of the brain.

- Back pain is rarely the result of an injury, but rather is something that comes and goes like a headache.

- There's a great difference between back pain and disability from back pain.

- The brain can create pain or enhance pain through the nocebo effect.

- The brain can relieve or lessen pain through the placebo effect.

CHAPTER 3

THE ANOMALY AND ANATOMY
OF THE BACK

MOST core strengthening programs—and there are a lot of them out there—are designed to strengthen the abdomen with the goal of achieving a "six-pack" or losing inches off the waist. I'm going to push you to prioritize the actual *back* muscles, which turn out to be more important than the abdominal muscles when it comes to back pain. The Hidden Core Workout teaches you that you've misunderstood the term *core*, thanks to popular uses of the word by trainers who focus on ripping the muscles in the abdomen at the front of the body. Core work is not solely about the abdomen—quite the contrary. You will learn how to alter your posture and form by "locking" your back. This will require strengthening of your back muscles.

What the Hidden Core Workout does is build *all* of your muscles to form an internal brace around your entire core—front, sides, and back—similar to the rigid external brace you might see a worker wearing at Home Depot. This internal brace supports and immobilizes your back. It does this by first overemphasizing the hidden muscles in your back.

What if I told you that the exercise system in the Hidden Core Workout trains the core muscles and develops them in such a way that you build an internal brace that locks and protects your back *while also minimizing belly fat and a creating a six-pack*?

Well, hold onto your central nervous system, because I just did!

Hidden Truth 8: Look in the Mirror and Ignore What You See!

Alternatively, you could take every mirror in your house and throw them out the window. But what I really mean by this paradox is that you should change your motivation for strengthening your core. Most of us construct an exercise routine as a reaction to what we see in our full-length mirror, if we have the guts to look long enough (or at all). Who doesn't want visible abs? Couple that with the fact that we hear about how integral core strengthening is to having a healthy back, and it's confusing to know where to place your priorities.

What do I mean by this? Wouldn't the widely touted core strengthening accomplish both? Not unless you're practicing the program of the *hidden* core. This is because, simply put, the core ab work typically done to achieve a six-pack works only on "superficial" muscles. The Hidden Core Workout tackles muscles that are deeper than the visible muscles on the surface—and, more importantly, the muscles that are behind you and not seen in the mirror. It's these hidden core muscles that are the foundation of the internal brace mentioned above.

Roth's R$_x$: Build your *hidden* core as opposed to the muscles you see in the mirror, and you'll not only help your back pain, but you'll like what you see in the mirror as well!

In chapter 1, I discussed the wonderfully adaptive capability of both the brain and the body. You're going to learn how to utilize this capability and actually change your back (and your brain). In order to implement the program, you'll need to have a basic understanding of bending, core anatomy, and how building an internal brace will affect your posture and form.

THE NOT-SO-SIMPLE ART OF BENDING

Weight lifters can squat or deadlift enormous amounts of weight. They're not born with this natural ability; they have to learn how to "lock" their back and pelvis during a lift. This is accomplished by a combination of muscular tone, ligament strength, and tightening of connective tissue in conjunction with the development of an "awareness" of technique. These adaptations can be developed by following a simple series of exercises and by willingly adopting a particular "form" while bending or lifting. Learn the following equation:

$$\text{Posture} + \text{Form} + \text{Awareness} = \text{Core Strength}$$
$$P + F + A = C$$

How we hold and maneuver our bodies requires mastering a dynamic between gravitational pull and muscular action. When we're standing, the term *posture* is applied to this dynamic. When we're exercising or performing tasks, the term *form* is applied. In both settings, the dynamic between gravity and muscular action is mediated "cognitively" by *awareness* and "physically" by *core strength*. Posture and form thus arise out of the synergy between the brain and body.

Awareness starts with understanding that when you bend, you have a choice between bending your *back* and performing the same task with your back straight and "locked," which is done by rotating your

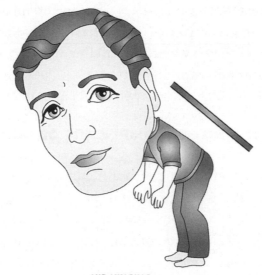

HIP-HINGING

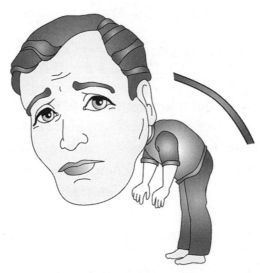

BACK-BENDING

pelvis forward, a movement known as *hip-hinging*. It's important to understand that hip-hinging is the safer of the two options.

Go to the mirror (yes, that dreaded mirror) and observe yourself bending your back. Then compare that with bending by hip-hinging. The first thing you'll likely notice is that hip-hinging requires back strength; it's hard to maintain your back locked in a straight position while you bend. The second thing you'll notice is that your hamstring muscles tighten as you go down, limiting your range of motion. The more flexible the hamstrings are, the lower you can bend down with a straight back (that is, by hip-hinging). This is the ultimate goal. The Hidden Core Workout develops both strength and hamstring flexibility to facilitate this protective locked form and motion.

Returning to the example of weight lifters, would you be surprised to learn that they're one of two groups of Olympians least likely to injure their back? (The other group, which should come as little surprise, is table tennis players.) This may seem counterintuitive, but it makes sense when you consider weight lifters' obsession with form in conjunction with awareness, preparation, and core strength.

Along these same lines, the men and women who move luggage in airports often say that large suitcases that are actually empty and light cause them the most trouble. If a suitcase is predicted to be heavy, and it *is*, there's less risk for injury. If a worker anticipates a load to be heavy, however, and it turns out to be light, his or her form will be potentially compromised, which can cause an unexpected movement, with subsequent injury to the back or its musculature. In that case, the lack of awareness, more than the weight, is what causes a problem.

One other important area that should be stabilized during bending and lifting is the sacroiliac joint. In order to stabilize that joint, the brain automatically rotates the sacrum (the last bone of the spine) anteriorly relative to the pelvis (a move known as nutation, addressed

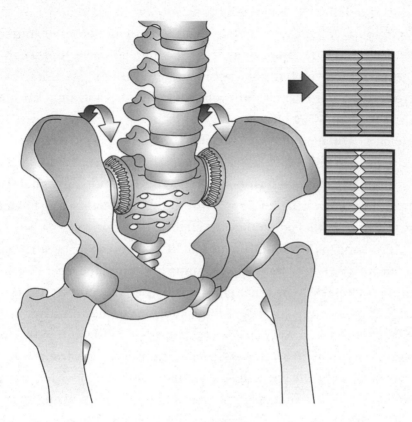

SACROILIAC JOINT:
THE ARROWS SHOW NUTATION.
THE JOINT CAN BE "LOCKED" BY PUSHING THE PELVIS INWARD TOWARD THE SACRUM.

below) and pushes the two halves of the pelvis (the ilium bones) toward the sacrum.[1] Both actions "lock" the sacroiliac joint so that motion is eliminated between the sacrum and the pelvis.

Don't worry about this complex move—it becomes automatic as you learn to lock your back.

Let's put all the motions together now. Don't worry: I'll keep it simple.

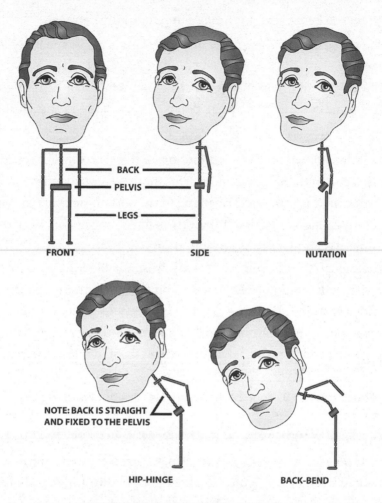

BACK-BENDING, HIP-HINGING, AND NUTATION

Think of your body, when you're standing, as consisting of three separate structures stacked on top of each other. On top is the spine. Under the spine is the pelvis. Under the pelvis are the legs.

Each of these structures is free to move relative to its adjacent structure, as if via hinges. The spine can move relative to the pelvis, for example, and the pelvis can move relative to the legs.

When you bend, several things can potentially happen:

- The top structure, the spine, can bend. This is what I mean by *back-bending.*
- The pelvis can tilt on the legs. This is what I mean by *hip-hinging.*
- The spine can also tilt on the pelvis. This is done at the sacroiliac joint.

As noted above, the forward motion of the sacrum relative to the pelvis occurs at the sacroiliac joint. This motion is called nutation, from the Latin word for "to nod," referring to the sort of rocking that's seen with a spinning gyroscope. When the sacrum moves backward, the movement is known as counter-nutation.

The hidden part of your core is also responsible for tightening the sacroiliac joint and thus keeping the spine locked into the sacrum. As we move ahead and discuss posture, we have to remember not only how the spine should be oriented, but how it should be oriented relative to the pelvis and how the pelvis should be oriented relative to the legs.

Hidden Truth 9: Your Back Should Be Straight When It's Bent!

This concept will gradually be incorporated by your brain, and then by your body (or vice versa). It's one of the central tenets of this book. If you can learn to keep your back straight and hip-hinge rather than back-bend, you'll protect your back and limit pain. You should practice this posture and form over and over again so that it becomes habitual.

First, though, in the rest of this chapter, you need to learn a little anatomy.

Roth's R$_X$: Learning how to bend and how to pick up objects with hip-hinging rather than back-bending is key to a healthy back. With practice, this will change your posture and your form and decrease your back pain.

POSTURE ANALYSIS

Did you know that your head weighs about eighteen pounds? Most of us never feel that weight because it's balanced on the top of our spine. However, anyone whose posture or balance is thrown off knows how heavy the head can feel. Try walking around with your head flexed forward, or with your whole back flexed forward like Groucho Marx. You won't make it for even five minutes without neck or back fatigue and pain!

With altered posture, the necessary increase in the supporting muscles' workload often results in back pain. Pain can also arise from asymmetric stress on supporting structures. One of the many reasons that patients have persistent back pain is that their posture is altered during the acute phase of the pain. Even after the original stimulus has healed, the altered posture and pain can persist.

In a normal (or what we call "good") posture, the head is balanced on top of the spine, which is balanced on top of the pelvis. The pelvis is then balanced on the legs.

There are, however, four common variants of posture, all of which disrupt the spine's natural line of gravity. To compensate for any of these disruptions, the body tries to regain balance. Under normal posture, the spine has an *S*-shaped curve to it that's balanced over a line of gravity. The following four irregular postures affect that *S* shape. Let's take a closer look at each one.

1. *The sway back:* In this posture, the pelvis is held in *front* of the sacrum. Also known as lower cross syndrome, the sway back is the result of the pelvis being thrust forward without actually tilting. This posture, found in many patients with back pain, is increasingly seen in our culture of excessive sitting. The key to improvement of this posture lies in the strengthening of the gluteus muscles and the hip flexors.

2. *Hyperlordosis:* This posture is similar to the sway back, but there's more inward curvature (lordosis) in the lower back and the pelvis is tilted forward. This posture is seen in many obese patients. Treatment consists of abdominal and gluteal muscle strengthening and hamstring flexibility training.

3. *The flat back:* This is nearly the opposite of the lordotic—naturally curved—back. Lordosis is absent in the lumbar spine, and the pelvis is tilted posteriorly. This is seen in patients who've spent time doing only anterior abdominal exercises such as crunches. Treatment requires strengthening the hip flexors and multifidus muscles and stretching the hamstrings and abdominal muscles.

4. *The kyphotic back:* In this posture, the shoulders roll forward and the thoracic (middle) spine curves forward. This is more a problem of the upper back musculature, with weakness of the scapula stabilizers. The condition is treated with back strengthening, with particular focus on the upper back muscles, such as the rhomboids

Lower Cross Syndrome

Lower cross syndrome was discovered by Vladimir Janda, a physician with a keen interest in postural imbalance. He identified a subset of patients with a swayback posture who he thought had probably ended up with this posture because of excessive sitting. Swayback patients develop tightness and shortening of the hip flexor muscles (the psoas major, the iliacus, and the rectus femoris) and consequent lengthening and weakness of the "crossed" muscles (the gluteus maximus, gluteus minimus, and gluteus medius). These people develop back pain in part because of the constant back muscle contraction needed to counter the abnormal posture.

(major and minor) and the trapezius, multifidus, and serratus anterior muscles.

In each of these four variants, irregular (or "bad") posture can become chronic. Some muscles and supporting ligamentous structures can shorten, while the opposing muscles and supporting structures lengthen and weaken. Treatment to improve posture must, therefore, come in stages. The first stage is awareness. The next stage is a combination of stretching and strengthening to correct the shortened and lengthened structures, respectively. The final stage is practicing until the change is ingrained.

YOUR BACK ANATOMY—A BEGINNER'S BREAKDOWN

As an overview, your core has an anterior (front) component, a posterior (back) component, and two lateral (side) components. Each of these components has a superficial and deep layer. The anterior, lateral, and posterior components are connected to each other by fascia (strong connective tissue) to form a "belt."

The Visible Core

Let's get into a little more detail by starting with the more familiar core muscles.

Anterior superficial muscles: These muscles are "superficial" in that they're the muscles that lie just beneath the skin. Technically, the ones in the front are called rectus abdominis, (*rectus* meaning "straight"). The rectus abdominis muscles form two vertical masses down the anterior wall of the abdomen. In between is a midband of connective tissue. When these superficial muscles are worked, they, along with the vertical midband between the muscles, become visible, assuming there isn't a lot of belly fat.

Anterior deeper muscles: If the rectus abdominis muscles are superficial, something has to be underneath, deeper, right? Of course. And in the front, we call those muscles transversus abdominis (*transversus* meaning that the fibers of these muscles run horizontally).

Lateral muscles: The internal and external oblique muscles are lateral—that is, located on the sides of the abdomen. These muscles are involved in side bending and twisting.

Now think of this varied group of muscles working together: When the rectus abdominis (anterior), transversus abdominis (also anterior), and obliques (lateral) are worked properly, and there's an absence of belly fat, a visual six-pack is produced.

While a ripped stomach is what most people want, studies have shown that programs that isolate only this section of the abdomen can cause an asymmetry that may actually weaken the back. That's why the Hidden Core Workout focuses on continuing the strengthening program *around* the entire back—like a brace, as noted earlier, or the body's natural weight-lifting belt.

The Hidden Core: An Overview

We have many muscles that make up the core other than the ones mentioned above, but they're the forgotten ones. As a society, we're concerned with, and influenced by, only things that we can *see*. To ignore or neglect the body's "hidden" muscles is as logical as dyeing the gray out of just the front of your hair. Just because you can't see what the back or inside of you looks like doesn't mean you want to ignore it, right? The same concept goes for developing the hidden core.

So what *is* behind you? And what are the interior muscles that you can't see? In short, what is the hidden core, exactly? The good news is that getting to the backside of you isn't as futile as a dog chasing its tail; the bad news is that you'll have to read through a bit more of my back "breakdown" to get the information you need.

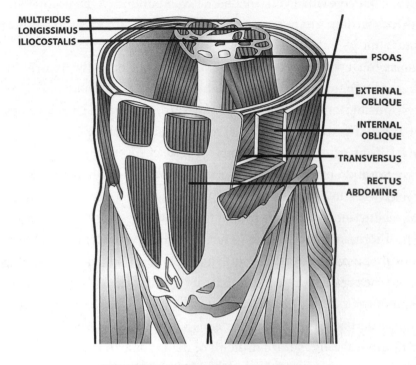

FRONT VIEW OF THE SUPERFICIAL AND DEEP BRACES

Before we get to specifics about individual muscles, let's take a big-picture look: Technically, the core muscle group at your back is referred to as the posterior core or the posterior chain (*posterior* meaning "behind" or "at the back"). These muscles, in combination with the visible core muscles described above, complete the internal belt or brace that we'll build using the Hidden Core Workout in chapter 4. The posterior muscles are connected to the anterior and lateral muscles, thanks to a connective fascia. When all of the muscles are contracted—front, back, sides—this fascia can be tightened to "squeeze" the abdomen and stiffen the spine. This tightening effect is facilitated by a "hydraulic amplifier," whereby the fluid in the tissues is com-

pressed. It's like when you squeeze a water balloon in the middle and the ends stiffen. That's your *entire* core working together to support your spine.

Remember the brace image I left you with earlier? Now picture this brace as *two* braces, one inside the other. The outer (or superficial) brace is responsible for moving your body forward, backward, and sideways, while the inner (or deep) brace serves as a stabilizer, keeping your back still while another part of the body moves.

An example of the stabilizer effect can be seen when you watch bicycle riders from behind. I remember watching a televised analysis of two elite riders who were filmed from behind as they raced against each other in a sprint. Ultimately, one of the two riders was able to maintain more speed despite equivalent pedaling speed and pedaling power. The commentator concluded that the slight sway back and forth of one of the riders allowed for a loss of energy. The rider who could stabilize his back while still moving his legs maintained greater speed. You might imagine that it's difficult or defies logic to keep your spine still while moving your legs vigorously. It would, except that the posterior chain, when developed, is responsible for stabilizing the spine itself, and holding the spine to the pelvis during movement.

That point is worth restating: The inner brace not only stabilizes the spine itself; it also locks the spine to the pelvis by keeping the sacroiliac joint stable. The Hidden Core Workout is all about developing the posterior chain of muscles, in particular, in order to allow for this stability (and the subsequent reduction in back pain).

Are you ready for the next level of complexity? The superficial and deep braces are further strengthened by muscles that can pull those braces up and down. All of the primary core muscles work in conjunction with other muscles that are both superior (higher, toward the head) and inferior (lower, toward the pelvis). The core is pulled toward the head by the pectoralis and serratus anterior muscles, which are located in the front of the body, and by the latissimus dorsi muscles, which are

located in the back. The core is pulled toward the feet by the psoas muscles and the quadriceps femoris muscles (in front), and by the gluteus maximus muscles (in back). Think of your core as your belt and these other muscles as your suspenders, pulling the brace up and down as needed.

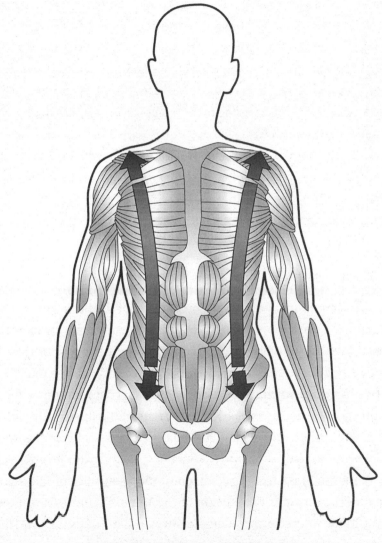

"SUSPENDERS" PULL THE HUMAN BRACE UP AND DOWN.

Core Concept
||||||||||||||||||||||||||||||||||||

I hope you can see now how core strengthening addresses all three potential causes of pain: painful stimulus, epiphenomenon, and the brain's judicial function. First and foremost, the hidden core stabilizes the spine and fixes it to the pelvis, thereby reducing motion of the spine. Second, the hidden core strengthens the muscles and the fascia themselves, which helps reduce pain in these structures. Third, the hidden core influences the judicial function of the brain, because the more you change your reaction to pain from a lack of movement to a movement using your tightened core, the more you perceive pain and treatment differently. By pushing yourself out of your normal thought processes, you alleviate the fear, anxiety, and lack of knowledge of pain that caused your false interpretation of pain in the first place—a biological bait-and-switch.

The Hidden Core: What Does What

We're just about finished with our breakdown of the back. However, we still have the posterior muscles to learn. Although we've seen their general function, we now need to address their specific duties. The superstars of the neglected hidden core are the multifidus muscles.

The posterior core muscles have a superficial component called the erector spinae muscles, which are composed of the iliocostalis, longissimus, and spinalis muscles. This superficial muscle group gains its power by its increased distance from the spine (greater leverage), but the unique orientation of the deeper multifidus muscles provides more than half the power for extension of the spine. In addition to power, the multifidus muscles provide stability and, more importantly, the ability to individualize movement of the spine on a segmental basis.

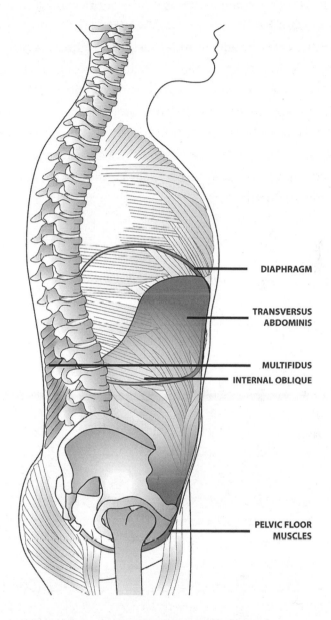

DIAPHRAGM

TRANSVERSUS
ABDOMINIS

MULTIFIDUS
INTERNAL OBLIQUE

PELVIC FLOOR
MUSCLES

THE MULTIFIDUS MUSCLES AS PART OF THE CORE TEAM.

In other words, the unique anatomical configuration of these muscles can control the movement, not only of the entire spine, but of any two individual segments of the spine. Think of the larger muscle groups as being able to move the whole spine like the straightening of a bent rod, while the multifidus group is able to individually straighten a bent chain. This allows for each individual vertebral body to interact with its neighboring bodies separately from the gross movements of the whole spine.

To understand why the multifidus muscles are so special, we need to know their unique anatomy. The muscles connect the rearward tip of each vertebral body (known as the spinous process) to the facet joints and the thoracolumbar fascia.

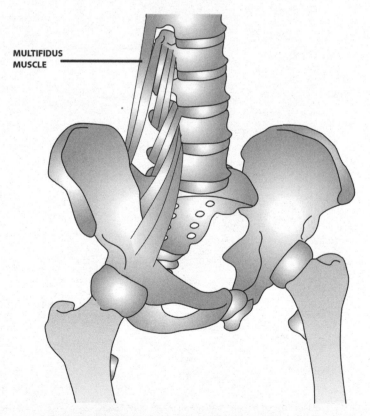

MULTIFIDUS
MUSCLE

**PART OF WHAT MAKES THE MULTIFIDUS MUSCLE SO SPECIAL AND SO ABLE TO
PROVIDE STABILITY IS ITS VARIETY OF DIFFERENT ATTACHMENTS.**

Though the terminology may be daunting, you're on intimate terms with the actual body parts: The spinous processes are the bones that you feel through the skin on your back when doing sit-ups on a hard floor, the facet joints are the paired joints that allow for flexing and straightening the lower back, and the thoracolumbar fascia is part of the internal belt or brace described earlier in this chapter.

This anatomical arrangement allows a multifidus muscle to use the spinous process as a lever arm or a handle for moving each vertebral body. Because it's attached to this longish handle, the muscle can exert a relatively large amount of torque for its size.

Its attachment to the capsule (or surrounding layer) of the facet joint puts tension on the capsule so that when the spine is extended, that capsule is pulled and tightened, and thus not "pinched," as the joint goes through its motion. (Pinching of the capsule is a potential source of back pain.)

Similarly, the muscle's attachment to the deep fascia, or connective tissue, allows it to help tighten the deep transversalis fascia and thus tighten the inner brace described above.

Finally, its attachment to the pelvis aids in the stabilization of the sacroiliac joint.

Electromyography (EMG) tests, which can measure the electrical activity of muscles, have revealed several interesting findings about the multifidus muscles. In cases of disc herniation, for instance, an injured nerve can atrophy, or weaken, the multifidus muscles through disuse or denervation. This weakening of the multifidus muscles is directly correlated with back pain. In other words, one interesting and largely unrecognized way in which a herniated disc can cause back pain—as opposed to the obvious way that it can cause leg pain—is by weakening these muscles.[2]

An easy way to improve back pain from a herniated disc, then, is to improve function in the multifidus muscles. The way to do that is through exercise.

> ## Core Concept
> IIIIIIIIIIIIIIIIIIIIIIIIIIIIIIIIIII
>
> If you remember one thing about the multifidus muscles, it should be this: They provide about 70 percent of the stiffness of the spine during straightening up from a bent position. In other words, if you develop your multifidus muscles, your spine should be able to remain relatively stiff when you move. This will minimize back pain. By strengthening these hidden core muscles, you not only complete a tightening brace that immobilizes the back and helps you bend and keep a healthy posture that eases tension from the back, you also immobilize and protect the vertebrae of the lumbar spine and avoid the pain associated with pinched nerves, herniated discs, and other painful back ailments.

Abnormal EMGs of the multifidus muscles have also been found in patients with focal spinal instability, or laxity between two adjacent bones, a condition known as spondylolisthesis. In this condition, one bone "slips" forward on the adjacent bone. Although this condition sometimes require the bones to be fused together, strengthening of the multifidus muscles has been shown to reduce pain. Exercise and strengthening of these hidden core muscles have been shown to improve both the pain and the EMG of the muscles. MRI studies also correlate atrophy of the multifidus muscles with chronic back pain.

In short, there is anatomical, electrical, and radiological evidence that links multifidus functional loss with back pain. Recovery of this muscle function with exercise will decrease back pain. This is true with herniated discs, postsurgical back pain, spondylolisthesis, and back pain due to pregnancy.

As special as the multifidus muscles are, like all great performers they have a supporting cast:

- Gluteal muscles
- Quadratus lumborum muscles
- Psoas muscles
- Hamstring muscles

Gluteal muscles: Collectively known as "the glutes," or "the muscles of the butt," the gluteal muscles consist of the gluteus maximus, gluteus medius, and gluteus minimus. The gluteus maximus is the largest and most superficial of the three. Since the gluteus maximus has its origin in the sacrum (the large, triangular bone at the base of the spine) and the ilium (the uppermost and largest bone of the pelvis), it connects the spine and pelvis to the leg. Given that linkage, it's both a powerful stabilizer of the pelvis to the spine and an extensor and external rotator of the hip.

The gluteus medius and minimus are smaller and deeper muscles that push the legs away from each other. Because of the gluteus maximus's helpfulness in stabilizing the spine and pelvis, which enables hip-hinging, you'll find that the exercises in the Hidden Core Workout particularly incorporate strengthening of the glutes in addition to the other muscles of the posterior chain.

Quadratus lumborum muscles: The quadratus lumborum are paired muscles that connect the ribs to the pelvis and also connect to each transverse process (the portion of each vertebral body that juts out laterally). They serve as guy wires, so to speak, in supporting the spine to the pelvis. Interestingly, it's nearly impossible to walk without these muscles, as they provide the stability to allow each leg to be lifted during walking. These muscles are essential in maintaining posture during the transfer of weight.

Psoas muscles: The psoas muscles originate in the front of the spine and descend over the pelvic brim to connect to the legs. If the spine is fixed, the psoas muscles flex the hip. When a person is standing, the psoas muscles pull the lumbar spine anteriorly, helping to promote a normal curvature. Although the psoas muscles don't insert into the pelvis, they cross the pelvis and thus function as another pelvic stabilizer.[3]

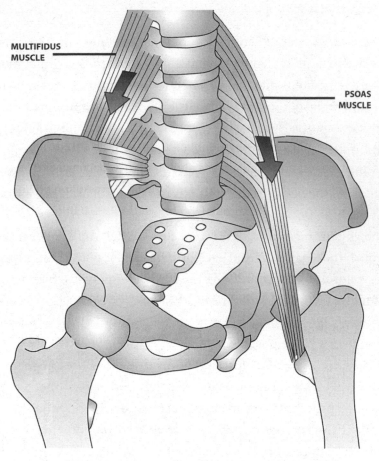

MULTIFIDUS
MUSCLE

PSOAS
MUSCLE

DEPICTION OF THE MULTIFIDUS AND THE PSOAS MUSCLES WORKING TOGETHER
TO STABILIZE THE LUMBOSACRAL SPINE AND ITS ATTACHMENT TO THE PELVIS.

Hamstring muscles: The hamstring muscles are much more than just the leg muscles that flex the knee. Each hamstring muscle is actually three separate muscles: the biceps femoris, the semimembranosus, and the semitendinosus. This three-part muscle crosses the hip joint

Focus on Philosophy
||||||||||||||||||||||||||||||||||||||||||||||||||||||||

The Frankl Principle

Viktor Frankl was a neurologist and psychiatrist who applied some of the existential principles of philosophy to the discipline of psychiatry.[4] His unique experience of being a concentration camp survivor likely helped shape his philosophy, which focused on finding meaning in the face of difficult circumstances. I include two quotes from Frankl:

"When we are no longer able to change a solution, we are challenged to change ourselves."

"Between stimulus and response there is a space. In that space is our power to choose our response. In our response lie our growth and our freedom."

The Frankl principle is thus the idea that we have to adapt in difficult situations that we can't change—like some experiences of pain. This principle involves understanding the difference between what life gives us and what we make of what life gives us. In the world of pain, many patients go through a transition from trying to understand where the pain is coming from to learning to deal with the pain. This is an example of the Frankl principle.

as well as the knee joint. It serves as a hip extender and provides stability by adding a resistive force when hip-hinging.

Hamstring tightness is commonly seen in patients with back pain. This makes sense, because the tighter the muscle is, the harder it is to hip hinge (and thus the more a patient needs to back-bend when bending forward).

Now that you've seen the relevant anatomy, I hope that you're convinced of the need to build yourself an internal brace. Before giving you the exercise program that will help you do that, I'll go over some general concepts that will provide for you a handy philosophical guide. As much as you may be tempted to skip to the actual exercises, you must be willing to take responsibility for your own pain, and that involves some additional learning.

The Hidden Core Workout automatically helps to correct most postural abnormalities. You'll learn specifically why and how this is true in the next chapter, where we'll transfer our focus from the question of "What's wrong with me?" to "How do I get better right now?"

This answer is, simply, "With action."

The Gist

- Strengthening your back and learning how to hip-hinge rather than back-bend is essential in treating and avoiding back pain.

- Your body has a circumferential built-in brace that can be strengthened.

- Strengthening the brace will improve most cases of back pain.

- The brace is comprised of three parts—anterior, lateral, and posterior—each of which has a superficial and deep component.

- The core is composed not only of this brace, but also of the supporting muscles that pull the brace up and down (the suspenders, if you will).

- The "hidden core" is both the most important and the most overlooked part of the core. It consists of the important multifidus muscles, the superficial erector spinae muscles, and a supporting cast of muscles that include the glutes, the quadratus lumborum, the psoas, and the hamstrings.

CHAPTER 4

THE HIDDEN CORE WORKOUT

THE HIDDEN CORE WORKOUT is an exercise program that you can customize to fit your pace and confidence level. In as little as six weeks you can radically improve your back health and strength. Continued use of the program will then maintain back health and reduce the incidence of back pain. If you need more than a week to feel comfortable moving from one step to the next, take it. This program is a slow and steady approach that will instill lasting change.

This is a stackable program, meaning that each week you add more exercises to your workout. The program is specifically designed to build strength, working your back muscles first, to catch up to your more developed abdomen. As you gain strength, the program focuses on developing the muscles of the imaginary brace, as well as the "suspenders" that pull the hidden core and anterior wall vertically.

Ideally, your exercises should be done three times a week, or every other day. Your body will tell you when you've had enough, but it's important to understand the difference between pushing your body out of its comfort zone and causing damage. Don't be afraid to stretch a little longer, or go for another repetition ("rep"), as long as your form is correct. If you feel that you're sacrificing form in order to get through another rep, *stop*. If you continue beyond that point, you will only slow your progress by having to take time off to recover.

FROM ISOMETRICS TO MOVEMENT

The Hidden Core Workout was developed to strategically build the muscles of the posterior core, as well as the more familiar abs, to complete the internal brace illustrated in chapter 3. Workout participants accomplish this through graduated exercises that progress from isometrics (which by definition are done in a static position) to exercises of motion.

As discussed earlier, there are three potential causes of back pain: a painful stimulus (including movement), an epiphenomenon (usually in the form of immobility, muscle spasm, or postural change), and the judicial function of the brain. With movement contributing to the pain problem, you start the Hidden Core Workout with exercises that build the muscles while isolating them with isometric training—not with exercises that require range of motion. As the muscles of the Hidden Core strengthen and your brace develops, you then graduate to range of motion exercises that increase stamina and work the abdomen in conjunction with the back. The result: better posture and a decrease in back pain.

STRENGTHENING BEFORE STRETCHING

Stretching and strengthening of the muscles must be done together. Many therapy programs involve *only* stretching, but isolated flexibility programs can leave patients susceptible to injury. In the initial acute state of pain, particularly, flexibility should not be sought until strength and endurance have been initiated. It's amazing how often I've asked patients if their physical therapy involved strengthening and they responded yes, but when I asked for specifics it was clear that all they did was stretch. There's a difference between stretching and strengthening, and while you need both, you should start with strengthening.

ENDURANCE OVER MAXIMAL STRENGTH

In the Hidden Core Workout, strengthening is focused more on endurance than on maximal strength, since the aim is to change your posture. This is achieved by higher repetitions targeting "slow-twitch" muscles, the stabilizing muscles that are related to posture and endurance. Another way of thinking about this, anatomically, is that the bulk of the early strengthening will be isometric (as noted above), without a lot of range of motion, and will target the deeper, stabilizing muscles.

The previous chapter's discussion of muscle physiology revealed a complex array of muscles that perform a variety of tasks. But don't worry: You won't have to remember all of these muscles. The Hidden Core Workout is divided into six stages, or "weeks," targeting the appropriate muscles at the appropriate time. Perform and complete each week as you see fit for your level, but don't forget the Nietzsche principle, which encourages you to put up with some pain as you progress.

You must trust that your body is naturally designed to coordinate your muscles, leaving you to focus only on your form. I urge you to work out until fatigue limits your ability to perform with good form. In other words, don't jerk the last few repetitions to get to an arbitrary number. Let your body work out the functional coordination of its muscles on its own. Your job is to focus on movements, not on muscles.

As is the case with many attempts at dieting, lots of people experience a brief loss of willpower followed by a more prolonged abandonment of the program. Just as success in dieting requires the acceptance of occasional straying from the routine with a quick return to the diet, so too is the case with this exercise program. You *will* miss days and you *will* have setbacks. The key is to get back on the horse and try again.

The Primal Human
||||||||||||||||||||||||||||||||||||||||||||||||||

There has been a popular return to "primal" considerations in terms of our nutrition, psychology, biology, and so forth. In diet and nutrition, so-called paleo adherents are proponents of returning to the nutritional and physical habits of our cave-dwelling ancestors, claiming that our biological needs have not evolved over time and are not equipped to process the prepared foods and lack of mobility that permeate our culture today.[1] This primal idea has been extended to our habits of exercise and to a rise in interest in evolutionary psychology, with simple yet sensible ideas to fix our harried lifestyles—by allowing sunrise and sunset to determine our sleep patterns, for instance, or by eating only foods that are in season.

This same argument can be extended to the treatment of back pain. Trusting in our primal instincts, we would rationalize that the body knows how to properly engage its processes and repair itself, if allowed to function as it biologically and instinctively knows how—that is, through movement. Our ancestors certainly had no time for bed rest or even significant time to heal, but rather must have developed ways to get better while maintaining an active pursuit of food. After all, getting food was a life-or-death matter. If you stopped *moving,* you didn't find food and starved, or shelter and froze, or a mate and . . . well, you know.

Heck, you could have been eaten!

When rest of different durations has been compared to simply trying to return to activities of daily living, the latter effort yielded far better short-term and long-term control of back pain. Trust your body's ability to recover and be resilient. Your ancestors couldn't afford to rest, and neither can you!

GETTING STARTED

The only equipment needed for the Hidden Core Workout is a kettlebell and an exercise ball (a fifty-five-centimeter ball if you're under five foot eight and a sixty-five-centimeter ball if you're five foot eight or taller). Both these items can be bought at any sports gear store.

The recommended kettlebell starting weight for men is *approximately* thirty pounds. (Stronger-than-average men can increase that, and weaker-than-average men should definitely decrease it.) For women, the recommended kettlebell starting weight is approximately twenty pounds, which also can be increased or decreased, depending on strength. If you're not sure, always start with a lighter weight. Older patients, and people with no experience with kettlebells, should always start with a lighter weight. It's always better to start lighter and slowly increase the weight over time. Form is paramount and should dictate kettlebell weight. I would suggest that you peruse YouTube or professionally done videos that can help with your form.

HOW KETTLEBELLS WORK THE HIDDEN CORE

I know what you're thinking: If I'm expected to lift weights, why doesn't the Hidden Core Workout utilize traditional dumbbells? The kettlebell's center of mass (unlike that of the dumbbell) is extended beyond the hand, which facilitates the swinging of the weight with added safety and added grip, wrist, arm, and core strengthening. The result is that you can lift, bend, squat, and even perform deadlifts with more ease and less risk of injury using kettlebells.

Most kettlebell exercises require the kettlebell to be picked up off the floor. This forces you to be aware of proper posture, while simultaneously stretching and strengthening the hamstring muscles. In a kettlebell swing, the pelvis rocks forward and backward on the legs

What's a Kettlebell?
||||||||||||||||||||||||||||||||||||||||||||||||||

The kettlebell has been in existence for more than three hundred years and is thought to have originated in Russia. It's a cast-iron weight resembling a cannonball with a handle that allows it to be swung.

Kettlebells can be bought in pounds, in kilograms, or in a Russian measurement called a *pood* (equivalent to about thirty-five pounds, or sixteen kilograms). The various swinging exercises done with kettlebells in the Hidden Core Workout work the entire body—in particular, the back.

Kettlebells—or *girya,* in Russian—provide an aerobic function in addition to their back-strengthening and hamstring-stretching roles. Kettlebell swings are said to burn about twenty calories per minute, or the equivalent of the calories expended by a person running at a sub-six-minute-mile pace!

Research has shown that heart rate and VO_2 score (which measures delivery of oxygen to muscles) can be improved with kettlebell training. That these are markers of aerobic capacity underscores the power of kettlebells to provide both strength and aerobic benefit.

A group of subjects was tested using a standard battery of physical tests, including pull-ups, jumping, running, and sprinting. Part of this group was then given a standard exercise program designed to increase the results on each of the tested areas. The other part of the group was instructed to undertake a kettlebell workout. When the two groups were retested, the kettlebell group performed with better results than the group that had worked a standard exercise program.[2]

When overweight people work out with kettlebells, their weight drops, and when thin people work out with kettlebells, their muscularity increases!

through the hip joint. This action is mediated primarily by the gluteal muscles and the hamstring muscles. The strengthened gluteal muscles are then more capable of stabilizing the pelvis to the spine by immobilizing the sacroiliac joint.

While the body goes through this motion, the spine must be held stiff. This requires engagement of the multifidus muscles. Similarly, holding the spine stiff through a ballistic (swinging) motion engages the entire core, which simultaneously tightens the internal belt, utilizing the hydraulic amplifier, as discussed above.

That's a lot going on, right? Throughout your workout, the swinging motion of the kettlebell forces the brain to coordinate the relative contribution and timing of these various components of the posterior chain through a variety of different positions.

Much back pain occurs only with motion. I've previously discussed the benefits of performing activities that *can* cause pain, but doing them in a painless way. That approach utilizes the science of embodied cognition. Swinging the kettlebell with proper form epitomizes the idea of successfully performing a motion that one would think would be painful.

What makes kettlebells unique is that the handle allows for *swinging* the weight. You probably think I'm completely off my rocker, telling a person with back pain not only to lift but then to *swing* a kettlebell! By now, though, you know that I'm a sucker for a good paradox. This is yet another hidden truth. The ballistic motion of a kettlebell swing requires the constant engagement of the posterior chain of muscles through a range of motion. Posture and form *must be* maintained or injury is likely to result, which forces an awareness of form and posture. After practice and time, the body will adapt to this new form and posture, eventually making them second nature.[3]

Similarly, after a few workouts you'll start to incorporate your new posture and form into your work, play, and other activities of daily living. Then next time you go to lift your kids' toy trucks off the floor, you might find yourself hip-hinging without even thinking about it. Need to take out the garbage? You might find yourself in a slightly lordotic position as you lift the can. Pushing that heavy upright vacuum cleaner underneath the couch? You might not be hunched over. You might find that you sit down and get up differently or exit the car more efficiently, using your stronger glutes and hamstrings, which takes the pressure off the spine and back, alleviating pain naturally.[4] And guess what? In *all* cases, you'll find that your back doesn't hurt as it used to. All because you took on the self-efficacy of your treatment as well as taking a leap of faith in the kettlebell.

BREAKDOWN OF THE HIDDEN CORE WORKOUT

Week 1: Exercises 1 and 2

Week 2: Exercises 1 through 4

Week 3: Exercises 1 through 7

Week 4: Exercises 1 through 10

Week 5: Exercises 1 through 12

Week 6: Exercises 1 through 13

Beyond Week 6: Choose among exercises 1 through 12 and increase the repetitions of the Kettlebell Swing; consider adding the Burpee and the Turkish Get-Up (14 and 15).

Before and after each workout, do a warm-up and cool-down. I've offered some sample stretches for these purposes.

On the days you take off, I recommend either walking or running, or a combination of both. Don't be afraid to run if you have a bad back. I find that alternating the core exercise program with aerobic exercise allows the core muscles time to recover and adds the benefits of aerobic exercise.

Focus on Philosophy
IIIIIIIIIIIIIIIIIIIIIIIIIIIIIIIIIIIIIIIIIIIIIIIIIIIIIIIIIII

The Sartre Principle

Jean-Paul Sartre wrote about our tendency to label ourselves and then subscribe to the self-labeled behaviors. For example, calling ourselves lazy can become a justification for behaving in a lazy fashion. He believed that this tendency is rooted in the desire to escape from the existential burden of our actions. Instead of deciding to act lazily, we act that way because we *are* lazy—or so we tell ourselves. I call this the Sartre principle. The message is that we can be or do what we want, and we bear the full responsibility for that decision every day.[5]

Hidden Truth 10: "Walking Is Better Than Running" Is *Back*ward!

"Walking is man's best medicine," said Hippocrates over two millennia ago. Walking has been prescribed by doctors as a treatment for obesity, depression, and sleep disturbances (among a myriad of other ailments), generally as an alternative to medication. In patients who have back pain, the advice is often expanded to include the cautionary disclaimer: "Walk, don't run. The pounding is no good for back pain."

While I agree that walking is therapeutic for many ailments,[6] I believe that running offers even more benefits than walking. I make it a habit to scrutinize the MRIs of runners who visit my office. Over the years, I've been impressed at the condition of their discs: They're remarkably well preserved. This is no accident. There are studies that compare the spines of female gymnasts and female nongymnasts of the same age and weight. The spines of the gymnasts appear younger and less degenerated than those of their nonactive counterparts.[7]

For the most part, running is protective of back health. The only patients I discourage from running are those with severe degenerative disc disease and/or a history of consistent back pain when trying to run.

Interestingly, the book *Born to Run* by Christopher McDougall explores the relationship of running injuries to the "advances" of running sneakers. Citing two studies that compared barefoot and shod runners, he suggests that increasing the padding on the heel, for example, contributes to a style of running that lands on the heel rather than the ball of the foot, and is therefore more likely to cause back pain or injury.[8] This same concept can be applied to the spine, where wear and tear may serve to protect rather than to harm.

In those cases of degenerative disc disease where there may be a risk to "pounding" or wear and tear, the transformation from a style of running that involves the "heel strike" to a technique that involves landing on the front of the foot is advised. This form, as evidenced in barefoot running, has been shown to transfer less stress and thus be gentler on the spine. (One caveat: Although gentler on the spine, it may be harder on the feet.)

Humans evolved over millions of years to travel, work, and acquire food using two legs. Over the past 150 years, there has been a drastic change in our habits, with much more time spent sitting. This sedentary lifestyle has undoubtedly had a negative effect on our aerobic condition, back muscles, and general health. The incorporation of more walking—and, ideally, running—is a perfect antidote to many of our health issues, including back pain.

Roth's Rx: For most people, running isn't bad for the spine, but is actually beneficial. For those few who don't tolerate running well, altering the style of running to eliminate the hard heal strike may help. Finally, if you can't run, walk.

How do you know if you're making progress? How do you know if the program is succeeding? For some, the back pain will decrease. For others, the program will simply improve the ability to tolerate pain. The most common finding, however, is that the frequency, duration, and intensity of setbacks decrease. This may take months to occur, but the results will be long-lasting.

Warning: You may start to love your mirror and what you see in its reflection!

Hidden Truth 11: You're Smarter Than Your Doctor!

I'm eighty-six and my doctor used to tell me to slow down—
at least he did until he dropped dead.

—CESAR ROMERO

Personally and professionally, I believe in the effectiveness of the Hidden Core Workout, but it, like most programs, must be individualized to some extent. Blindly adhering to a program is nearly as dumb as trying to make one up without any experience. Remember the Maugham principle: Sometimes it takes more strength and character to *change* than to *persevere*.

Often, a disclaimer is made in books like this one, advising readers to "consult with your doctor before starting this program," but that implies that your doctor knows for sure whether the program is safe for you. This sort of legal disclaimer always makes me laugh. I'm a doctor who has studied this subject intensively, and I don't believe that *I* have all the answers, never mind *your doctor,* who may not have any experience at all with exercising for back pain (or with exercising, period)!

This doesn't mean I won't disclaim my own book on its copyright page (I do) and again right now by encouraging you to ask for your doctor's advice. I do remind you, however, to bear in mind that your physician is giving you an *opinion*. You can never know in advance if a particular routine will succeed or fail, and allowing someone else to make a guess about it is not what this book espouses. Rather, it's up to *you* to take the bull by the horns and decide if this (or any other) program resonates with you.

Roth's R$_x$: The Hidden Core Workout is worth a serious try. I've seen many skeptical patients embody both the Kierkegaard principle and the Maugham principle: They take a leap of faith and try something new, ultimately believing that they have nothing to lose. After a period of strengthening, most of these patients go on to improved back health and never look back.

WEEK 1

1. YOGA CAT STRETCH

Purpose: This is a warm-up exercise that directs blood supply to your back and core muscles.

Starting position: Get on your hands and knees on an exercise mat, with your knees directly under your hips and your wrists directly below your shoulders, fingers pointed forward.

Action: Exhale as you tuck your tailbone down and use your abdominal muscles to round your back and push your spine toward the ceiling, while rolling your shoulders forward. Allow your neck to lengthen and your head to reach down toward your chest. Hold for three seconds.

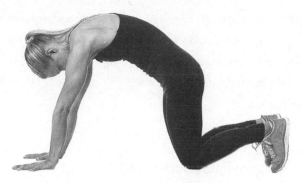

Now reverse the position by inhaling and using your abdominal and lower back muscles to lower your abdomen toward the floor. Tip your tailbone up toward the ceiling as you roll your shoulder blades back and together, lifting your head up slightly. Perform this sequence three or four times.

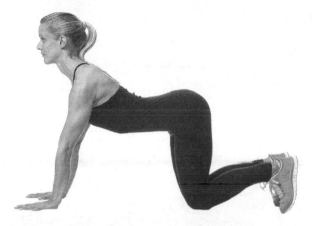

Coaching keys: Perform this move slowly, without any sudden movements. Repeat the sequence three to four times; you should be able to stretch a little farther each time.

What you strengthen: While this isn't a strengthening exercise per se, in that you're not building muscle tone through this stretch, you're encouraging flexibility, which is helpful to prevent injury when it's time to strengthen. More important, in this case, you're recruiting blood supply to your back and therefore are warming up. Focus and breathing, when combined with a proper stretch, can do wonders to prepare you for a solid workout.

Goal: As you go through this exercise, try to stretch a bit farther each time, visualizing your spine reaching even higher toward the ceiling and, in the reverse position, your abdomen lowering to the floor. Each time you challenge yourself, try to feel some heat going into your back as blood supply is increased.

2. KNEELING SWIMMER'S STRETCH

Purpose: This exercise strengthens your back and serves as a warm-up.

Starting position: Get on your hands and knees on an exercise mat, with your knees directly under your hips and your wrists directly below your shoulders, fingers pointed forward.

Action: Tighten your abdominal muscles to stabilize your spine. Keeping your head in a neutral position, simultaneously extend your left arm in front of you until it's parallel to the ground and extend your right (opposite) leg until it's also parallel to the ground. Keep your spine and head aligned; don't allow your back to sag or arch.

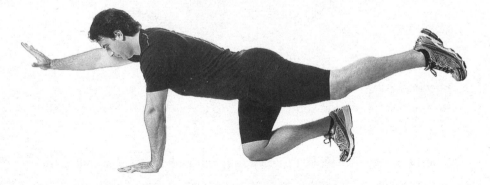

Hold this position for two seconds and then return to your starting position. Repeat, reversing the position with your right arm forward and your left leg pointing backward, keeping your spine in a neutral position throughout. As noted above, any exercise program has to be tailored to the individual; thus I won't specify reps. Simply repeat this exercise (and subsequent exercises) as many times as you can do so without losing form.

Coaching keys: This exercise should be done slowly and in one continuous motion. The exercise can be made more difficult by holding each rep for a slightly longer amount of time. This will help to improve endurance.

Alternative 1: If this move causes shoulder discomfort, support your upper body on a chair or exercise ball and perform only the leg extension.

What you strengthen: This exercise works the muscles that support the spine (sometimes called the paraspinal muscles), including the multifidus muscles, the erector spinae muscles, and the gluteal muscles.

Goal: The aim here is to develop your balance and endurance. Feel the muscles in your back as they're being targeted. Your shoulders and your buttocks will be used as well. Try to fully extend your arm and leg on each repetition.

WEEK 1 RECAP

Once you've done three sessions of the above two exercises, which will take you around one week (given your days off), add exercises 3 and 4 so that your routine now includes four exercises. It's reasonable to spend another week with week 1 if you're sore or believe that you're not ready to move on to week 2.

Your anterior core is most likely stronger and more developed than your back muscles. That's why the Hidden Core Workout works only your back muscles initially. That lets them catch up to the strength of your front abs.

WEEK 2
||||||||||||||||||||||

With this week and subsequent weeks, only the *new* exercises are mentioned. You'll begin, though, by doing previously mastered exercises (as outlined in "The Breakdown of the Hidden Core Workout").

3. FRONT PLANK

Purpose: This is an isometric anterior core exercise. It will strengthen your abdominal muscles without putting your spine through a range of motion.

Starting position: Lie on your stomach on an exercise mat with your elbows close to your sides. Slowly, lift your torso off the floor or mat, your weight divided between your forearms and feet. Keep your back straight by contracting your abdominal muscles.

Action: Simply hold the final position while breathing normally for ten seconds to start, adding time as you become stronger.

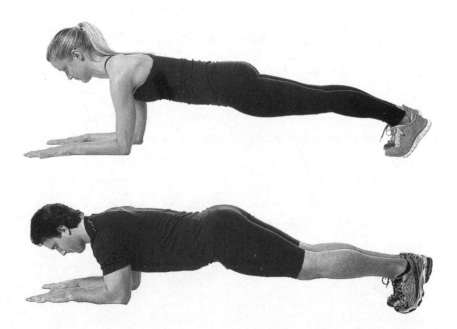

Coaching keys: Stop if your hips begin to hike up or drop down, or if you're otherwise unable to maintain the proper form. If you experience back pain, lift your hips slightly.

Alternative 1: If the position hurts your shoulders, do this exercise on an exercise ball. "Hug the ball" rather than support yourself on your arms. Easier yet is to lean against the wall (rather than lying prone) and support your weight with your forearms.

Alternative 2: Start out in the original position but support your lower weight on your knees rather than your feet. That will make the exercise easier.

What you strengthen: The exercise works the rectus abdominis muscles, oblique muscles, and transversalis muscles.

Goal: Focus on keeping your body straight. The goal is to shorten the distance between your rib cage and your pelvis.

4. SIDE PLANK

Purpose: This exercise isometrically strengthens the lateral part of your core: the internal and external obliques.

Starting position: Lie on your side on an exercise mat and prop yourself up on one elbow and forearm, keeping your other arm straight down to

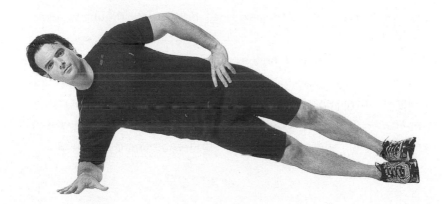

your side or with your elbow bent and your hand at your waist. Keep your legs unbent with your feet stacked on top of each other. Contract your abdominals and raise your hips off the ground until your body forms a straight line. Don't let your hips drop.

Action: Simply hold the position (breathing normally) for ten seconds to start, adding time as you become stronger.

Coaching keys: Stop if you're unable to maintain proper form.

Alternative 1: If this position hurts your shoulder, you can support the side of your upper body on an exercise ball rather than supporting yourself on the ground.

Alternative 2: Support your weight on your knee rather than your foot. That will make the exercise easier.

What you strengthen: This exercise is good for your internal and external oblique muscles.

Goal: Focus on keeping your body straight. You'll feel the muscular fatigue in the side that's closer to the ground.

WEEK 2 RECAP

Once you've been doing the above exercises (all four of them) for one week, you're ready to add the next three, bringing the routine to seven exercises.

You've been strengthening the anterior, lateral, and posterior core (the hidden core). Your focus thus far has been on isometric strengthening. The posterior core has now had (at least) two weeks to develop, laying the groundwork. The next phase, the three new exercises, will involve more range of motion and stretching while the strengthening continues.

WEEK 3
||||||||||||||||||

5. KETTLEBELL SQUAT

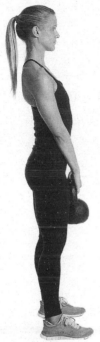

Purpose: This is an exercise that works the back, the buttocks, and the legs. It's a more functional exercise than those that you've done thus far, as it will prepare you to lift objects off the ground during your activities of daily living. This squat engages the core through the whole range of motion of the exercise. You'll notice that it may make you short of breath, because it requires many muscles to work at the same time.

Starting position: Stand straight, with your arms relaxed and in front of you, holding the kettlebell with both hands. Your feet should be shoulder-width apart, turned outward slightly, toes pointing to the ten o'clock and two o'clock positions.

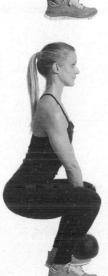

Action: Keep your shoulders drawn back and your back straight. Squat down by bending at the hips and knees, pushing your butt out and keeping your heels on the ground. Keep your eyes straight ahead as you lower yourself until your thighs are parallel to the ground (or until your heels start to come up off the ground). Return to the starting position by pushing through your heels. Avoid rolling onto the balls of your feet.

Coaching keys: Keep your shoulder blades pulled together and avoid bending forward. This enables the natural curvature of your spine (lordosis) to stay in a constant position. (For a review of posture and lordosis, refer to chapter 3.) If you experience knee pain, modify the movement by squatting halfway down (or however far you can get within a pain-free zone).

Alternative 1: In place of a kettlebell, substitute a large book.

What you strengthen: You'll work the multifidus and erector spinae muscles, the quadriceps muscles, and the hamstring and gluteal muscles.

Goal: Despite the fact that this exercise appears to focus on the legs, the act of maintaining your back posture is your main goal. If you have bad knees and don't want to squat too low, that's fine. Focus entirely on holding your back stiff (in lordosis) and holding your shoulder blades back. Do as many reps as you can, but don't compromise form.

6. STANDING HAMSTRING STRETCH
(GOOD MORNING STRETCH)

Purpose: This exercise is designed to strengthen your back as you maintain posture while hip-hinging forward. (For a review of hip-hinging, refer to chapter 3.) This exercise will also stretch and simultaneously strengthen your hamstrings in their elongated position.

Starting position: Stand with your feet shoulder-width apart, your arms down to your sides.

Action: Keeping your legs and back straight with your knees slightly bent, push your butt back slightly as you bend forward at the hips, placing your hands on your knees, fingertips pointed toward your toes. Bend forward (without rounding your back) until you feel tension in your hamstrings, at the backs of your thighs. Hold for five seconds. Slowly return to the starting position and repeat for a total of five times, each time going a little farther and holding the posture for a little longer.

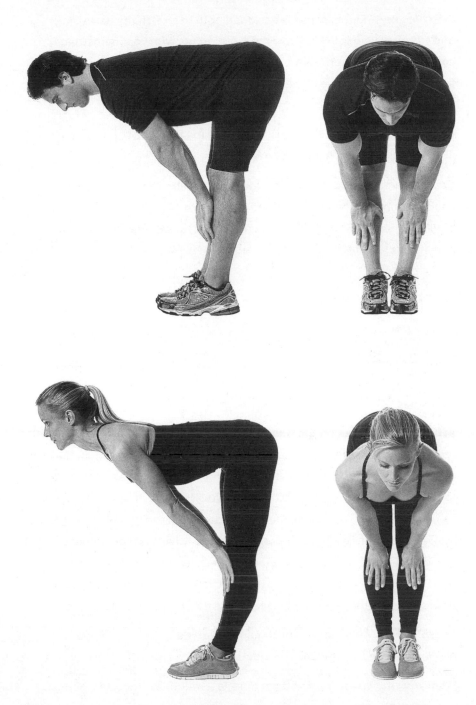

Coaching keys: This exercise is designed both to stretch the hamstrings and to help you practice the form of hip-hinging, with your hamstrings controlling the motion. Your body will gain the confidence it needs to hold this position. This is the one exercise you should repeat throughout the day—especially in the shower, when your body is warm.

What you strengthen: This exercise benefits the lower back muscles, gluteal muscles, and hamstring muscles.

Goal: As you maintain the stretch, focus on simultaneously arching your back and hip-hinging farther toward the ground. Keep your shoulder blades pulled back. Try to keep your back in lordosis while allowing your hamstrings to stretch.

7. YOGA BACK TWIST

Purpose: This exercise will stretch your hamstrings and your lower back and strengthen your obliques and your gluteal muscles.

Starting position: Stand with feet shoulder-width apart, your arms down to your sides.

Action: After performing the standing hamstring stretch (above) for five reps, add this movement: bend as if to touch your toes (a movement that requires back-bending as well as hip-hinging). Once you're as close to your toes as your hamstrings will allow, anchor your left arm on your thigh, your calf, or the ground (depending on how far down you can go). With your right arm held straight, extend it up and back, laterally twisting your upper body to the right. You may relax your left leg slightly as you twist to the right. Hold that right arm as far up as possible while looking as far up as possible. Repeat on the other side, holding each side for fifteen seconds.

Coaching keys: This movement should be worked into slowly. Keep pushing yourself to gradually twist farther.

What you strengthen: Your oblique muscles, multifidus muscles, gluteal muscles, and hamstring muscles are strengthened by this exercise.

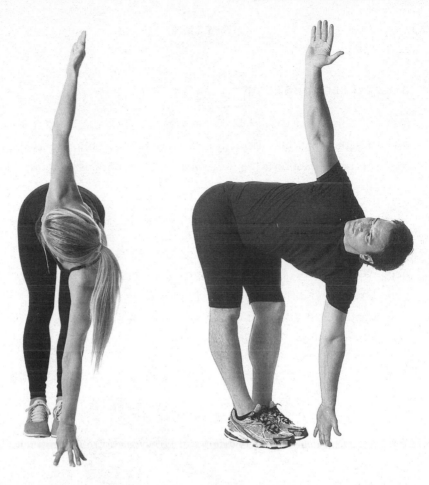

Goal: The goal of this exercise is to simultaneously stretch your hamstrings and strive for more twist in your lower back.

WEEK 3 RECAP

You've now finished a minimum of three weeks with the Hidden Core Workout and may be ready to add the next three exercises. This will make your routine ten exercises long. You've been doing isometric strengthening for the core, along with stretching and functional exercises. The next set of three are intended to add more function and range of motion and further target the anterior core.

WEEK 4
||||||||||||||||||||

8. KETTLEBELL DEADLIFT

Purpose: This exercise is similar to the Kettlebell Squat in that it uses many different muscles and may make you short of breath. However, a greater range of motion is required, which will strengthen your back. This is strictly a hip-hinging exercise.

Starting position: Stand with your feet hip-width apart, with the kettlebell on the ground between your feet.

Action: Engage your abdominal muscles and keep your knees slightly bent. Squeeze your shoulder blades together. Keep your back straight, hips slightly pushed back, as you bend forward at the hips (*not* the waist) and grab the kettlebell handle with both hands.

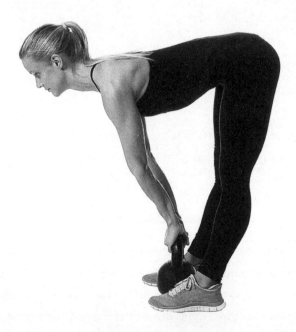

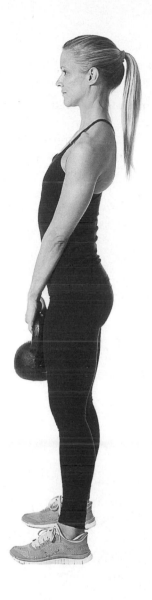

Pause slightly, making sure your heels remain in contact with the ground and your shins are parallel to each other. Keeping good form, raise back up to the starting position with your arms straight, bringing the kettlebell with you.

Coaching keys: If your hamstrings are tight, you may find it necessary to bend your knees in order to reach the kettlebell. Bending your knees causes you to use your back muscles more, while keeping them straight relies more on your hamstrings. The purpose of this move is to engage the back muscles, so slightly bent knees work best. Continue until you can no longer do the exercise with good form.

Alternative 1: Use a heavy book or just your body weight initially if the kettlebell seems too heavy.

What you strengthen: This exercise calls on the multifidus muscles, erector spinae muscles, gluteal muscles, and hamstring muscles.

Goal: Your aim here is to strengthen your back muscles while stretching your hamstrings and to practice proper bending techniques.

9. OBLIQUE V-UP

Purpose: The Oblique V-Up is similar to a sit-up except that you're not on your back, but midway between your back and your side. This oblique position shifts the focus from your rectus abdominis to the oblique muscles.

Starting position: Lie on your left side with your legs extended and your left arm resting on the ground next to your side, with your palm down. Cup your right hand next to your right ear. Roll your hips back so that your legs, still stacked, are at a slight angle to the ground. (Remember, you want to be lying midway between on your back and on your side.)

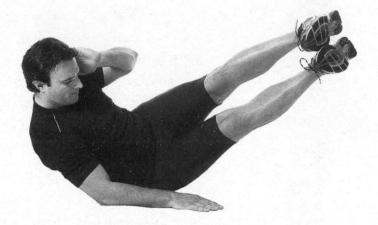

Action: Simultaneously lift your torso as you bring your legs off the ground and bring your right elbow toward your right knee. Repeat to the point of fatigue; then reverse sides.

Coaching keys: Avoid pulling your head or neck with your hand. Focus on using your core muscles to bring together your knees and elbow.

What you strengthen: This exercise works the oblique and rectus abdominis muscles.

Goal: Focus on maintaining balance in this oblique orientation and shortening the distance between the rib cage and the thigh.

10. HAMSTRING CURL ON THE FITNESS BALL

Purpose: This exercise will strengthen your hamstrings differently than the hip-hinging exercises, such as the Kettlebell Deadlift and the Standing Hamstring Stretch (Good Morning Stretch), because the knees will be bent for most of the hamstring contraction of this curl. Since the hamstring muscle crosses two joints (the hip and the knee), it responds differently when the knee is straight than when the knee is bent. In addition, this exercise will strengthen the anterior core.

Starting position: Lie on your back on a mat with your heels resting on the top of the center of the ball, toes up toward the ceiling, arms at your sides.

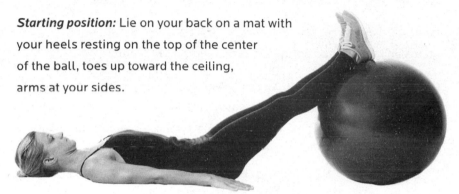

Action: Raise your hips until your shoulders, hips, and knees align; don't arch your back. Slowly bend your knees as you roll the ball (using your feet in a gradual pulling motion) toward your hips, without allowing your hips to drop. Pause and return the ball to the starting position; repeat without resting your hips on the ground between reps.

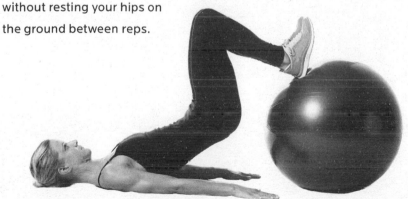

Coaching keys: Keep the core engaged by keeping your hips held high and not allowing them to drop as you roll the ball back and forth.

Alternative 1: If you don't have a fitness ball, place your heels on the seat of a sturdy chair or couch. Then lift your hips, keeping your body aligned from shoulders to heels, and hold your posture until fatigued. Gently lower yourself to the ground between reps.

Alternative 2: Do the exercise as described, but also lift your arms off the ground. This will require more core strength to maintain balance.

What you strengthen: You'll strengthen the transversalis abdominis, rectus abdominis, and oblique muscles with this movement.

Goal: Although this strengthens your hamstrings, it's primarily an anterior core exercise. Focus on lifting your hips as high as you can, and hold the position for a second at the end of each rep to make it more challenging.

WEEK 4 RECAP

You're now a minimum of four weeks into the program and are ready to add two more exercises, bringing your routine to twelve exercises. Your back and core should be feeling stronger and your hamstrings should be more flexible.

WEEK 5

11. BACK EXTENSION ON A FITNESS BALL

Purpose: This exercise strengthens the posterior core and puts the back through a range of motion.

Starting position: Kneel in front of a fitness ball and roll out on top of it until the ball is under your abdomen and your hands and feet are on the ground, your legs in a *V.*

Action: Keeping your hands on the ground in front of you for stability, bring your feet together and lift up your legs, squeezing your glutes and focusing on using your lower back muscles. Don't allow the ball to roll; keep your legs straight and your shoulders, hips, knees, and ankles aligned. Pause and hold the pose, and then bring your legs back to the starting position.

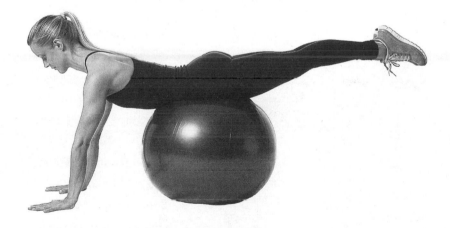

Coaching keys: Keep your motions smooth and controlled and focus on engaging the back muscles when your legs are at the highest point.

Alternative 1: If you don't have a fitness ball, try draping your body over a chair and follow the above instructions for lifting your legs.

What you strengthen: You'll feel a difference in your multifidus muscles, erector spinae muscles, and gluteal muscles.

Goal: Focus on lifting your hips and legs as high as possible without compromising your form.

12. BENT-OVER KETTLEBELL ROW

Purpose: This exercise will strengthen the posterior muscles of the upper back. Fortifying the abdominal "brace" requires building the "suspender" muscles that pull the brace toward the head: This exercise accomplishes that. Several of the previous exercises have worked on the glutes, which serve to pull the brace down toward the feet. By building the muscles that are above and below the abdominal brace, the brace is strengthened and the connective fascia, pulled in many directions, is tightened.

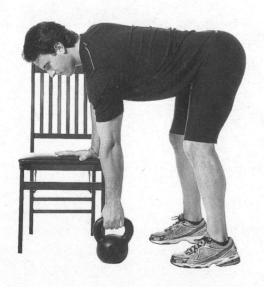

Starting position: Stand in front of a knee-high sturdy object such as a bench or chair and place a kettlebell between you and the bench or chair. Lean forward and place your left hand on the bench or chair, keeping your back straight and your feet flat on the ground. Your back should be parallel to the ground.

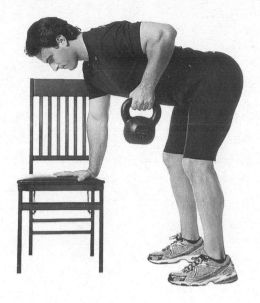

Action: While maintaining a flat back, contract your abdominals and grab the kettlebell smoothly off the ground with your right hand. Using a rowing motion, bring the right elbow up toward the ceiling; pause, and bring it gently down. Continue until you're fatigued or your form is compromised. Repeat on the opposite side.

Coaching keys: Focus on using your back muscles, not your biceps, to raise the kettlebell. This is done by constricting the shoulder blades.

Alternative 1: Use a book rather than a kettlebell.

What you strengthen: This exercise focuses on the multifidus muscles, oblique muscles, latissimus dorsi muscles, and rhomboid muscles.

Goal: Although this is an exercise that works on the arms and back, you should focus on elevating your shoulder blades, shoulders, and elbows rather than on bending your arms.

WEEK 5 RECAP

You are now a minimum of five weeks into the program and ready to add more complex exercises. The exercises to come will build on your current core strength and add an aerobic challenge.

WEEK 6
IIIIIIIIIIIIIIIIIIII

13. KETTLEBELL SWING

Purpose: This exercise forces you to stabilize your back and pelvis not only through a full range of motion in bending, but with a weight at the end of your arms that needs to be controlled continuously through its range of motion. This complexity forces you to engage the entire core throughout the exercise. This is an aerobically challenging exercise that will result in body fatigue and shortness of breath.

Starting position: Stand with your feet hip-width apart and with the kettlebell on the ground between your feet.

Action: Squeeze your shoulder blades together, keep your knees slightly bent, and tighten your abdominals as you bend forward at the hips and grasp the kettlebell handle with both hands. Lift the kettlebell by straightening your legs into the starting position. To begin the movement, push your hips back as you squat down, swinging the kettlebell back between your legs (keeping your back straight) and immediately swing it forward as you simultaneously straighten your legs and return to a standing position.

Extend the kettlebell forward until the arms are parallel to the ground at chest height. As you straighten your legs, squeeze your buttocks to engage the glutes. Repeat until your back is fatigued or you can no longer maintain proper form.

Coaching keys: Maintaining proper form is especially crucial for this exercise. Do the move in front of a mirror at first. Check out YouTube videos or seek professional instruction, if desired. This full-body move is actually a cardiovascular workout, because it works the back, hamstrings, and buttocks as well as the forearms. Strive to increase your reps over time.

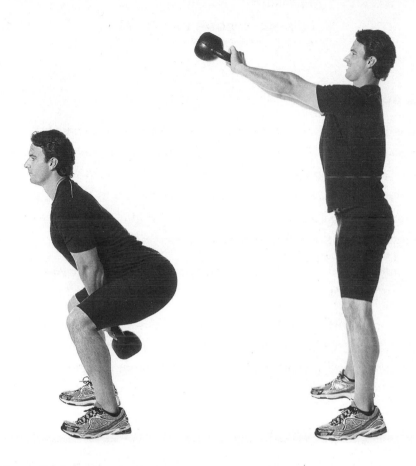

Alternative 1: Rather than a kettlebell, use a book.

What you strengthen: The entire core gets a good workout with this exercise. Although the hidden core is predominantly strengthened, the anterior and lateral core (along with supporting muscles such as the glutes and trapezius muscles) are also utilized.

Goal: Since this exercise can result in injury if not done properly, a premium should be placed on form. In particular, never allow yourself to relax the lordotic back position or the shoulder blade retraction. At the end of each rep, when the kettlebell reaches its highest point, snap the buttocks forward as if you were trying to squeeze a quarter between your cheeks.

ADVANCED CORE EXERCISES

|||||||||||||||||||||||||||||||||||||||||||||||||||||||||||||||||||||||||||||||||

14. BURPEE

Purpose: Like the Kettlebell Swing, this is a whole-body exercise that will fatigue you and make you short of breath. It requires engagement of the entire core throughout. Think of it as an advanced option. It's to be done only after the program has been completed and an adequate base of fitness has been built. The Burpee is technically difficult for older patients and should be used only by seniors who are exceptionally fit.

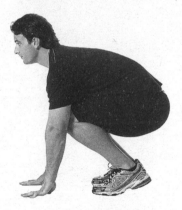

Starting position: Stand with your arms hanging down at your sides.

Action: Drop down into a squat by bending at the hips and knees and bringing your hands down to the ground in front of your knees.

Immediately raise your hips and kick your legs behind you, supporting your weight on your hands and, when your feet touch down, on the balls of your feet (as in a push-up).

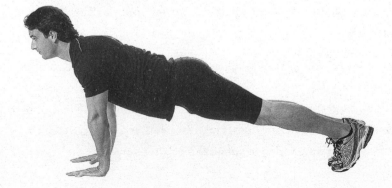

Next, with your weight on your hands, spring forward to return your feet to a squatting position. Finally, leap up, thrusting your arms above your head.

Coaching keys: Parts of this exercise are ballistic in nature. As difficult as maintaining form may seem, it is absolutely essential. Loss of form may lead to injury.

What you strengthen: The entire core and cardiovascular system get a serious workout.

Goal: This exercise will tire you after just a few reps. Don't lose concentration as you work through them. Try to add one more rep each time you go through this part of your workout, as long as you can do so without compromising form.

15. TURKISH GET-UP

Purpose: This is another whole-body exercise that requires full core engagement. Like the kettlebell swings and the Burpees, this exercise will leave you exhausted.

Starting position: Lie on your back with your left leg bent slightly and left hand pointed to the ceiling. (As you become stronger, hold a kettlebell in the raised hand.)

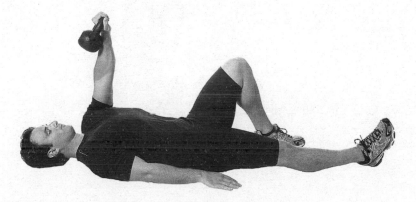

If you are holding a kettlebell, your grasp should be facing forward, with the kettlebell hanging over the back of your wrist and forearm.

Action: This involves several steps:

1. First, with your left arm pointed toward the ceiling, sit all the way up and place your right hand on the floor next to you.

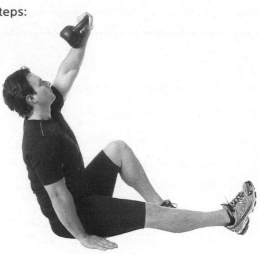

2. Next, swing your right leg so that it's behind you and you are supported on your right knee. Your left foot is on the floor while you continue to point your left hand toward the ceiling.

3. Finally, stand up gradually with your left hand still pointed toward the ceiling. (Imagine lifting a tray of glasses with that arm as you stand up.)

Now reverse the process:

1. First go down to the kneeling position with the left leg up.

2. Next, place your right arm on the ground and swing the right leg forward.

3. Finally, lie back down with the left arm pointed up.

Start with one rep on each side, then increase as tolerated.

Coaching keys: This complicated move, which requires balance and mental patience, is best learned by breaking it up into steps. Again, I would recommend watching a few YouTube videos. This is one of the most mentally challenging exercises you can do, because it requires maintaining intensity and focus for an extended period of time. It's great for eliminating asymmetries in your strength and form.

Alternative 1: If the kettlebell is too heavy, find a lighter object such as a book.

What you strengthen: The entire core is engaged throughout the exercise in order to maintain balance. The movement is also cardiovascularly demanding.

Goal: This exercise requires patience to learn and master. It also requires sustained concentration. Stick with it and you'll be mentally and physically tougher!

WEEK 6 RECAP

You have now completed the twelve exercises along with the kettlebell swings. At this point, you can continue to do the full workout three times a week or shorten the workout by omitting some of the earlier exercises and focusing on the exercises that seem to help you the most along with the more difficult and advanced exercises that are included: Burpees and Turkish Get-Ups. Never start with these exercises, as a warm-up is necessary to avoid injury.

The Gist

- The Hidden Core Workout must be introduced incrementally to avoid injury.

- The workout is based on exercise science and on the success that my patients with back pain have had with implementation.

- *Expect* setbacks. They're *not* an indication that the program won't work for you with time and dedication.

CHAPTER 5

DIAGNOSIS

A DIY GUIDE

WELL OVER two thousand years ago, Chinese general Sun Tzu said, "Know thyself, know thy enemy. A thousand battles, a thousand victories." We know those words today as a proverb describing the art of war, but it's a perfect summation of your personal war with pain. In diagnosing, treating, and battling pain, you need first to know yourself, and then to learn everything you can about your enemy—pain.

While *The End of Back Pain* focuses less on finding a diagnosis and more on searching for ways to mitigate pain, this chapter encourages you to learn as much as you can about the structures in your back that cause pain. Knowledge is power, yes; but as you now know, it's also a great contributor to self-efficacy and to mitigating the judicial function of the brain.

One important reason to seek diagnosis early is to uncover more serious conditions that can masquerade as common back pain. These conditions include tumors, infections, fractures, and serious inflam-matory conditions. You would, naturally, want an early diagnosis for these conditions. With that said, I intentionally placed this chapter on diagnosis *after* the exercise chapter in an effort to deemphasize the importance of diagnosis.

Remember, pain can be conceptualized as a triad—the stimulus, any resulting epiphenomena, and the judicial function of the brain. This chapter focuses on the original pain generator, the stimulus por-tion of that triad. You may be surprised to learn that the stimulus is unequivocally demonstrable in only a minority of cases.

Hidden Truth 12: Treatment Depends on Whom You See,
Not What's Wrong!

"If the only tool you have is a hammer, you tend to see every problem as a nail," said psychologist Abraham Maslow, and that assessment applies to today's options of diagnosis and treatment of back pain. For instance, when a patient presents to a healthcare provider with back pain, the treatment received depends more on where the patient starts his or her treatment than on the underlying condition responsible for the pain.

As a surgeon, I recognize that I'm in a discipline that's very much a part of the problem. I can't help but start my analysis of a patient who comes to me with back pain with the question, "Can I help this patient with surgery?" My true success as a surgeon, however, comes from transcending this bias. Although I have a hammer, I must look for things that are not nails.

So your back hurts. What do you do? Each healthcare provider car-ries inherent bias. If you ask a barber whether you need a haircut, what do you think that he'll say? Healthcare providers are *all* guilty of own-ing only a hammer (though the brand and style vary) and seeing only nails. Your starting point is terribly important because of this bias.

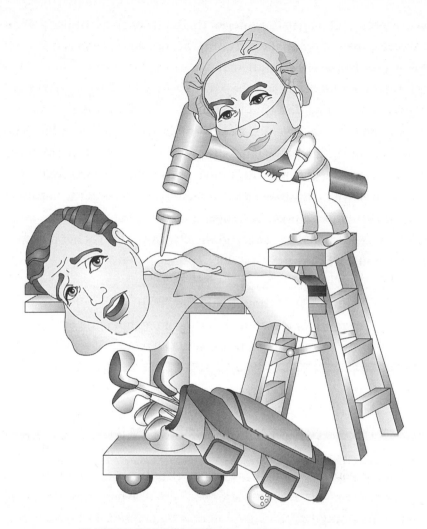

AN OVERZEALOUS SURGEON WHOSE ONLY INSTRUMENT IS A "HAMMER"

Consider the earlier-stated concept again: The caregiver that one sees determines the care that one receives more than does the underlying cause of the pain. How wrong this is!

One patient I treated, Diane, came to me after having been treated by a physical therapist for more than three months. Her chief complaint was intermittent pain in the anterior thigh that occurred mostly when she'd been sitting. Her pain had come on suddenly as she, a full-time nurse, was lifting a heavy patient.

I examined her and read the MRI. It showed a large, far-lateral, extruded herniated disc that the original radiologist had missed. I ordered an epidural injection of anti-inflammatory medication. The injection immediately alleviated Diane's pain so that she could begin to heal. Diane had started with a physical therapist, so the treatment she received was, of course, physical therapy. Because of the nature of her disc herniation, however, physical therapy was never going to work. Her treatment should have been guided by the nature of her disc herniation and not by the first practitioner that she saw.

Roth's R$_x$: Be careful where you start! You can't always know the correct starting point, but remain alert and ready to change direction.

THE REALITY OF BACK PAIN

Only about 30 percent of patients with back pain actually seek medical attention. Of those who do seek attention, about 90 percent will initially improve naturally over a two-week period. Remember, the body is naturally designed to heal itself. We now know that this improvement is not always complete, unfortunately; recurrence is more common than doctors previously believed. The good news is that less than 1 percent of conditions represent a serious or threatening problem.[1] That's not to say, however, that there's not an absolute need to uncover this 1 percent, especially given that many of these conditions will worsen or progress.[2]

There are a few commonsense factors that can help you determine if there's cause to believe you might be in this small minority: (1) If your pain is unfamiliar, it should be considered more than pain that you've experienced previously. (2) If you have a history of trauma, pain should be similarly red-flagged. (3) Finally, persistence or progression of pain is a sign to seek medical attention.

Recognizing a red flag is a touchy subject for healthcare providers, because the legal system looks *retrospectively* at the decision process, which puts healthcare providers in a legally vulnerable position. Given the legal ramifications, medical practitioners are conditioned to be so nervous about missing something that, even knowing how small the statistical chance is that there's something life-threatening about the patient, they order every test and screening imaginable, causing unnecessary anxiety and expense to the patient and the insurer.

Much has been written on the costs added to our medical system because of this legal burden. As long as healthcare providers are potentially liable for "missing" a diagnosis, there will continue to be an expensive and indiscriminant use of tests, so as not to miss a dangerous condition.

Trying to make a correct diagnosis insofar as it results in the best treatment is a worthwhile goal. However, often a definitive diagnosis is elusive, even with non-life-threatening problems. Still, seeing an expert early in the course of pain gives patients a sense of gravitas that serves to dismiss their worst fears of something "broken." This is exactly what happened with Tom, my suicidal patient mentioned in the introduction to this book, who called me in the middle of the night during my residency, and whom I talked off the ledge simply by debunking myths about his pain.

When you're suffering from back pain and trying to determine a course of action, it must sometimes feel like you're floating in the water with sharks circling around you. How can you protect yourself? First you have to try to figure out what's actually wrong. A precise answer may not be possible, but the more you can learn, the better. It's okay to see a diagnostician—in fact, I recommend it, as you'll see below—but only as a means for *you* to learn what's wrong. Remember, your health is *your* responsibility.

Hidden Truth 13: Start at the End, Not the Beginning—
Go Straight to a Specialist!

Trying to understand your condition early on is helpful. For that reason, I suggest that a specialist be seen early in your course rather than later, after the initial treatments have failed. I know that runs contrary to the conventional wisdom and may not be thought of as cost-effective. I would argue, however, that getting the diagnosis right *early* has the potential to save money. Remember Diane, for example, who went through several courses of unsuccessful physical therapy when an expert could have directed her to the correct treatment much earlier.

More important than an early diagnosis, moreover, is an early education. An expert can screen for the rare "red flags" that would signify a dangerous etiology for the pain. An expert can also identify what are now referred to as "yellow flags"—that is, personality subtypes or attitudes that suggest that the current pain may lead to a more chronic pain state.[3] Additionally, an expert can educate, dismiss counterproductive ideas, and help navigate you through the treatment process. Finally, the expert can help facilitate a transformation to an autonomous state, which is the key to ultimate back health.

Remember that the "right" diagnosis may not be forthcoming early in your course; in fact, it may never be conclusively made. That doesn't mean that you won't benefit from treatment. Often, the early diagnosis suggests that there's no definite cause for the pain. That's helpful, believe it or not, because it may serve to eliminate a lot of wasted treatments and future diagnostic "fishing" expeditions. A diagnosis of "no diagnosis" shifts the emphasis from "What's wrong?" to "What can I do?," which may be a good thing.

Even when no definitive answers are available at the outset, the diagnosis may become apparent over time. Paying close attention to how you respond to treatment can provide important diagnostic information. In other words, how you respond to any particular therapy may be helpful in defining what's actually wrong.

So can persistence. I had a patient come into the office for a third opinion. Cindy had originally experienced back pain and pain in her groin area. Two orthopedic surgeons had seen her, and both had recommended surgery on her spine. One had suggested a simple removal of a disc herniation, while the other had recommended a more complicated fusion procedure on her spine. She came to me because she was still not comfortable with the diagnosis, and she needed help deciding between procedures.

After careful examination, I concluded that her problem was not with her back at all, but with her hip. I redirected her to another orthopedic surgeon, who ultimately performed successful hip surgery that fully resolved her pain. I was impressed with her diligence; after all, not many people would seek so many opinions. She told me that her persistence was driven by a lack of comfort with the diagnosis. In particular, she was frustrated that the surgeons didn't "listen" to her and "just focused on the MRI" of her spine.

Once you start your quest for back pain treatment, it's essential to pursue an understanding of your condition and then, ultimately, to try to link that understanding with the correct treatment. It's also important to realize that this doesn't always work, or doesn't work right away; treatment is often a process rather than a single event. To a large extent, settling on the best treatment is your responsibility!

Roth's Rx: Take responsibility and try to figure out what's wrong, and then go straight to the expert. If you think your healthcare provider isn't listening, it's probably true—so move on and consult someone who *will* listen.

MEET MARILYN

Marilyn came into the office complaining of pain. When I asked her, "What hurts?" she answered, "My herniated disc."

When I then asked her, "What do you feel?" she answered, "My back hurts."

A patient who comes to the office complaining of pain from a herniated disc is a great example of how strongly some patients presume a cause for their pain and then link their pain to that cause. Marilyn's linking of her pain to the herniated disc that had been seen on her MRI by an earlier doctor is a natural and common response. Unfortunately, this sort of assumption often brings with it several other assumptions, such as "My pain will persist until the disc herniation is fixed," or "I'd better be careful with my activity, because I have a disc herniation." This is an example of the linguistic determinism that we discussed earlier. The diagnostic term "disc herniation" carries with it some heavy baggage. The mere *concept* of a herniated disc, whether such herniation exists or not, can actually do damage: It can create a disease and, as you've learned, actually lead to pain! (Just hold that thought for now. We'll return to disc pathology later in the chapter.)

It turns out that Marilyn had been having back pain for years. Her pain was present every day to some degree, but it was much worse if she moved or slept the wrong way. After one of her exacerbations, the pain would be much more intense for a number of days and then revert back to her baseline of low-grade, nagging pain. Marilyn had acquired the attitude and philosophy of avoiding activities that might "set off" her back pain. She had seen other healthcare professionals before me, one of whom had told her that she had "the spine of an eighty-year-old woman" and might "end up in a wheelchair one day."

Marilyn's presentation made it very clear that her chief complaint was based not on what she felt, but rather on what she'd been told—that she had a herniated disc. Her mind was centered, first and foremost, on having a herniated disc, with all the presumptions that logically followed. The verdict that she had an eighty-year-old's spine led to additional negative presumptions.

As her doctor, my first job was to disabuse her of her primary conviction, which was actually adding to her symptoms. It turns out that her "herniated disc" was no more than a typical sign of aging that's seen in many patients in their forties. The radiologist who first read the MRI had described one of her discs as herniated, a diagnosis that her internist had read and passed on to the patient. Yet another healthcare professional had looked at the MRI, and *he* told her that the reported diffuse degenerative changes were consistent with an eighty-year-old spine. Each of these statements was based on the assumption that the amount of pain and seriousness of pain could be construed by the findings on the MRI.

Because of these experiences, Marilyn was left thinking that because she had a herniated disc, she had a structural defect—a "broken" spine, in effect—and severe degeneration. Therefore, she believed that she needed to be "fixed" before she could resume normal activities and that, in the long run, she was in big trouble because her spine was aging faster than normal. Defeated, she believed that she might as well get used to limiting her activities.

I explained to her that what was on her MRI, while undeniably a disc herniation, could be seen in many women of her age who are asymptomatic, and that the MRI findings might have nothing to do with her intermittent exacerbations. Furthermore, restriction of activities would *not* alleviate the pain, I argued, but would instead contribute to back weakness and cause more pain.

When I examined her, she had only marginal weakness. Furthermore, her back was mildly tender to the touch, and she was unable (due to pain) to bend forward without supporting her back by putting her hands on her knees.

Ultimately Marilyn recovered with a combination of soft-tissue work (which consisted of massage, stretching, and heating) followed by aggressive back strengthening. "Recovery" in her case wasn't being pain-free, but being able to engage in most of her usual activities and having fewer exacerbations. When exacerbations did occur, she had the ability to self-treat and eliminate the symptoms quickly and without stopping her daily activities. Perhaps the true recovery was her escape from the mental burden of having "something wrong" with her spine. She accomplished this by utilizing the adaptive capacity of the back to improve her pain by actually *changing her back* through exercise.

JUST FIND ME THE DAMN PAIN GENERATOR!

By now you know my opinion about labeling your back pain, and you've heard the low odds that there might be something wrong with your back to the point where you need a specialist like me, need to alter your physical activities, or even need to have surgery. But luckily for me (and for the children I'm putting through college), there are times when there *is* a pathology that requires my diagnosis and treatment. So let's dig for that pain generator, even if it *is* a needle in a haystack, because you *could* be in that small percentage of people who have a problem that must be treated aggressively.

After I've completed the history and physical exam and have reviewed the MRI of a patient, I occasionally turn to more invasive diagnostic testing in an attempt to home in on the specific back pain generator, that good ole stimulus that we discussed in chapter 2. This is because an MRI, as we've seen, often shows many abnormalities that are simply normal wear-and-tear changes. It's a tough call, though: This more invasive testing can be problematic, painful, and far from perfect in its accuracy—it's fraught with both false positives and false negatives. Most importantly, it can be used to inappropriately justify treatments that are expensive and flawed in their efficacy. Despite these drawbacks, it's occasionally helpful to attempt to sort out which MRI abnormality is likely the source of pain.

This testing involves using a so-called live X-ray, produced with a fluoroscope, to place a probe into the exact area that the MRI suggests the pain seems to be arising, and then to either provoke the pain or try to relieve it. The decision to provoke versus relieve depends on where the pain is thought to originate. For example, discogenic pain is more easily provoked than relieved, while facet pain is more effectively relieved than provoked. An example of pain provocation is the discogram—a test performed by giving you brief sedation and passing a needle into a specific disc. Once you're fully awake, with the needles still in place, a clinician injects saline into the disc(s) in an effort to duplicate your pain. Does this sound barbaric? Well, it is! In addition to being barbaric, it's far from perfect. There are many times that a discogram suggests, incorrectly, that the pain is arising from the disc (false positive) or that the pain is not coming from the disc (false negative).

Still, I use the discogram on occasion, not as "proof" of a diagnosis, but as an additional piece of information to be considered with all the other information. It's essential that the person doing the test be impartial. Unfortunately, many discograms are done by a clinician who stands to benefit from a positive finding (since, for example, that finding might justify another treatment that the same clinician would do). If your doctor proposes a discogram as a diagnostic test to indicate a second procedure that he or she would do, I would suggest that you have the discogram done by another practitioner, one who doesn't stand to benefit economically from the ultimate procedure.

An example of a diagnostic test designed to *relieve* pain is the facet block, which also uses fluoroscopy. In this case, a needle is inserted, via live X-ray, into the portion of the facet where the nerve that transmits the pain from the facet is located. An anesthetic is then injected with the hope that the capsule of the facet joint will be denervated (that is, have its transmission of pain temporarily suspended) and the pain from that individual facet will be blocked. This test, too, is limited by inherent false positives and negatives and thus should also be administered by an impartial technician.

The provocative discogram and the relieving facet block are the two most commonly utilized invasive diagnostic tests for determining the cause of back pain. (More on such testing later.)

A DOWN-AND-DIRTY DO-IT-YOURSELF DIAGNOSIS

Are you ready for a quick overview of the identifiable causes of back pain? I'll make it simple—*overly* simple, in fact. This is just a rough guide. You need to understand that the process of pain identification is more of an art than a science. That explains why we can put a man on the moon and yet be unable to identify precisely where your pain is coming from—even after an MRI and a thorough history and exam.

Diagnosis can be tricky. It's tricky for me, and that's after twenty-five years of practice! I've already told you that most pain will simply come and go on its own, and I've suggested that of the pain that persists, most is not definitively diagnosable. In previous chapters I explained that pain may arise not only from a pain generator, but as a result of an epiphenomenon such as muscle spasm, postural change, or disuse. Finally, I've reinforced the idea that pain is always interpreted by the brain.

With all this in mind, let's start by looking at potential pain generators, but please don't discount the possibility of various epiphenomena or the interpretive role of the brain in creating, enhancing, or mitigating pain.

Conceptually, I divide back pain first into spinal and nonspinal origins. As a surgeon, I'm mostly concerned with spinal origins, which include things like herniation of a disc and arthritis of the spine. Nonspinal origins include muscular pain, pain arising from other support structures, and the nebulous concept of chronic pain (which, as we've seen, arises mainly in the brain). When I see a back pain patient for the first time, that's the first determination I try to make.

The next conceptual divide separates spinal-derived pain into discogenic pain and facetogenic pain. If the spine is looked at as a series of links stacked on top of each other, each link has an anterior part called the disc, and a posterior paired part called the facet joints ("paired" because there's one joint on each side), as shown in the illustration. (I'll explain the wheelbarrow later.)

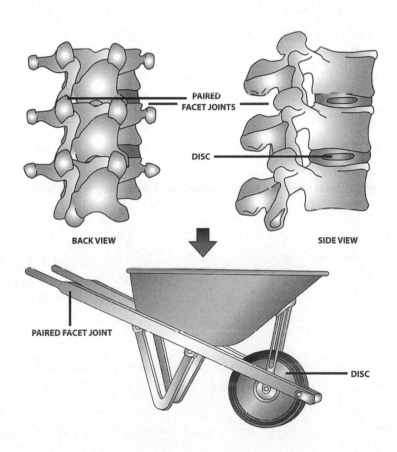

PAIRED
FACET JOINTS

DISC

BACK VIEW

SIDE VIEW

PAIRED FACET JOINT

DISC

While focusing on discogenic and facetogenic pain, I also keep in mind what's perhaps the most fundamental question of all: Is there an accompanying leg pain, and if so, what's its relative importance?

This differentiation of pure back pain from back pain with leg pain is essential. The addition of leg pain directly affects diagnosis, prognosis, and treatment. Later, you'll see that the pain generator can be more accurately defined in cases of back pain with leg pain. Additionally, the prognosis is better in those cases. Finally, because the cause of pain can more consistently be demonstrated in cases of back pain with leg pain, the treatment can be targeted. In such cases, I often hear myself saying, "The bad news is that you need treatment; the good news is that you need treatment."

With this background, let's begin the diagnostic process.

Is It a Disc Problem or a Facet Problem?

After you and any clinician(s) you've consulted have considered whether your back pain seems to be spinal or nonspinal in origin (a determination difficult even for a specialist), and whether there's leg pain or other leg sensation accompanying your back pain, you should consider how your back pain, and/or your leg pain, is affected by sitting, standing, and lying down.

This will help to distinguish between the two main players in the world of back pain: the disc and the facet. These two structures account for the majority of back pain in which a cause can be specifically identified, and thus it's important to learn about each of them. Bear in mind, however, that identifiable back pain makes up the minority of back pain.

In general, a problem with a disc will cause more pain in your back or leg when you're sitting and less pain when you're standing. In addition, lying flat on your back will likely be more comfortable than lying on your side. An issue with your facet, conversely, will generally cause more pain when you're standing than sitting, and lying on your side will be preferable to lying flat on your back. (I'll explain why in the next few pages.) Understanding that flexing the spine, or being in the sitting position, can aggravate the disc, while extending the spine, or being in the standing position, can aggravate the facet joints, underscores the potential for treating the pain by changing the posture.

We'll turn now to an overview of the disc and the facet. These are fascinating adaptations to the spine that allow, simultaneously, for strength and flexibility. As you might expect, however, this advantage comes at a price. The added mobility that these structures provide can be a source of pain.

Oh, My Aching Disc!

The disc is the largest avascular structure in the body (*avascular* meaning lacking blood vessels). It undoubtedly developed through evolution as a shock absorber for the spine. Without the disc being present between vertebral bodies, each step that you take would trigger a pain impulse to the brain from the impact of your feet with the ground. Interestingly, the shape of the spine itself also acts as a shock absorber. Rather than being straight, the spine has several curves that allow it to act as a Pogo stick: The spine's inherent "spring" prevents the impact of walking or running from generating a brain-directed impulse.

In general, herniated discs are found in younger patients. When we're born, the gel at the center of our discs is 70 to 80 percent water. As we age, we lose some of this water in a process called desiccation. It's while the discs are in their most water-filled state that we're most vulnerable to herniation. The discs themselves create height or distance between the vertebral bodies. This height creates tension in the ligaments that hold the vertebrae together. During the day, our discs lose water content and height. As we lose disc height, our spine can actually loosen up due to this loss of tension. This is why you should measure your height first thing in the morning. We all shrink throughout the day!

From the picture, you can see why sitting is painful for the patient with a herniated disc.

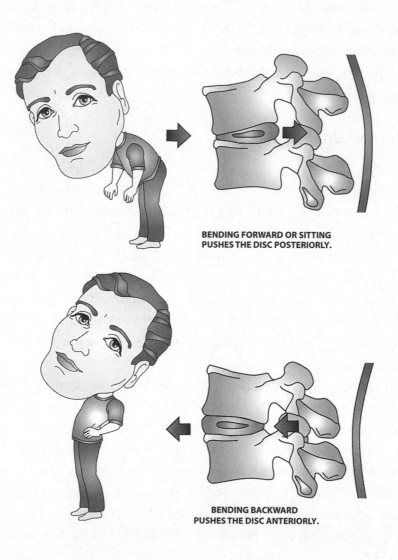

BENDING FORWARD OR SITTING PUSHES THE DISC POSTERIORLY.

BENDING BACKWARD PUSHES THE DISC ANTERIORLY.

> ## Core Concept
> |||||||||||||||||||||||||||||||||||||
>
> The herniated disc is a condition in which the gel that's the central portion of the disc tears the annulus, the surrounding outer layer. The terms *annular tear, disc bulge, disc herniation, disc protrusion,* and *sequestered disc* were likely coined to quantify how far the gel has migrated, but unfortunately, the terminology has no consistent use. If you're reading an MRI report, you can't draw any solid conclusions from the terms that are used.
>
> Since the nomenclature isn't consistently applied, you can't prognosticate based on the MRI report alone, even though how far the gel has traveled affects the prognosis, the type of therapy required, and the projected natural history. This is another reason to see a specialist relatively early in your course.

The flexed position of the spine that occurs while one is sitting (or otherwise bending forward) pushes the gel-like nucleus of the disc—more formally known as the nucleus pulposus—from front to back, stretching the circumferential surrounding ligament that holds the gel in (a ligament known as the annulus). That stretching or tearing ("herniation") causes stress on the annulus, which contains all the disc's pain fibers, or on the adjacent nerve root.

It's almost certain that you'll experience a herniated disc during your lifetime. Even if you're lucky enough to avoid this, you will certainly know someone else who has experienced it.

Is Your Disc at Risk?
The following facts must be considered when you're told that you have a herniated disc. I mention them here in hopes of helping you avoid negative outcomes that the diagnosis of a herniated disc often brings about—including inactivity, surgery, and/or hopelessness:

- Herniated discs are a common finding. MRIs done on asymptomatic patients often show herniated discs. In fact, the majority of herniated discs have no perceptible effect. Each decade in your life you'll likely accumulate more of these. So the first thing to remember is that if an MRI reveals that you have a herniated disc, it not only *may* mean nothing, it *probably* means nothing.
- Most herniated discs don't hurt.
- The presence of a herniated disc is relevant only when, in the minority of cases, that disc is the actual cause of pain. The majority of patients sent to me because their doctors thought that a herniated disc was the cause of reported pain turn out to have pain from a source *other than* the herniated disc.
- It's often hard to know if a herniated disc is causing the pain. This is why surgically treating the herniated disc doesn't guarantee that your back pain will be better. (That said, surgery *may* make the back pain better. However, it's very difficult to predict success.)
- Even once herniated, a disc doesn't always need treatment. The vast majority of disc herniations resolve themselves with time.

So, how do herniated discs cause pain? To answer this question, we must differentiate between how a disc herniation may cause *back pain* and how a disc herniation may cause *leg pain*.

Disc Herniation and Back Pain

Disc herniation may manifest only as back pain. I've already discussed one common cause of back pain as relating to the stretching or tearing of the annulus. Other possible causes of pain that disc herniation can trigger include loss of multifidus function, postural change, muscle spasm, and disuse of muscles and fascia caused by decreased activity.

If disc herniation *is* the cause of your back pain, how does the condition improve? Time. Physical therapy works in part simply by allowing time to work its magic. During that interval, targeted therapy strengthens the patient and helps mitigate epiphenomenal effects (such as postural change and spasm) and pain from lack of use.

Disc Herniation and Back Pain with Leg Pain

As discussed earlier, a key thing for you to consider is whether your pain is only in the back, or in both the back and the leg(s). If you have leg pain along with back pain, the exact location of the pain (or numbness or tingling) in the leg defines, in part, which nerve is being affected. The specific part of the leg works like a breadcrumb trail to lead you to the segment of the back from which the pain is coming.

This leg component is defined by the most distal (far away) aspect of the pain or other abnormal sensation. For example, if there's buttock pain and lateral thigh and calf numbness, the localizing component is the calf, because it's the farthest from the back. How does this "breadcrumb" effect work? Each spinal nerve root serves particular skin areas (called dermatomes) and muscle groups (myotomes). This means that identifying where the most distant localized pain is and which muscles are weak suggests which nerve root, and thus which part of the spine, is causing the pain. In other words, leg pain provides coexistent back pain with a "signature." When back pain is *not* accompanied by leg pain, the part of the back responsible for the pain is much more difficult to localize. (Later you'll learn about the various methods that we use to try to specify the anatomical cause of back pain when there's *no* accompanying leg pain.)

To understand how the spine/leg connection works, first picture the spine as a series of segments or joints. For example, L3–4 is the part of the spine that involves the bone called L3 (*L* for lumbar) and the bone called L4, along with the joints that hold these two bones together. Most of the time, back and leg pain arise from one of the three bottom spinal levels or segments, L3–4, L4–5, and L5–S1 (*S* for sacrum). If your pain radiates into the front of your thigh only, L3–4 may be a good bet. If the pain travels farther, into the bottom of the foot, then L5–S1, the bottom segment of the spine, is a good bet.

Coexistent pain in the leg and back doesn't arise simply from pressure on the annulus of the disc or on the nerve root. There must also be an inflammatory response. Because the disc's gel disc is avascular, it isn't exposed to the immune system, and thus, when it herniates and presses into surrounding tissue, it's viewed by the immune system as a "foreign body." As a natural defense to infectious or dangerous stimuli, inflammation sets in to initiate healing. Without inflammation, wounds and infections would never heal. This is the basis of the exuberant inflammation that often accompanies acute disc herniation. Ironically, when a person with disc herniation is given an epidural steroid injection, it's the inflammation that's targeted, not the herniation. (An injection can't alter the herniation itself.)

Surgery done on an awake patient demonstrates that a normal nerve root isn't sensitive to manipulation. Contrast this to a nerve that's inflamed: The slightest pressure can be excruciating. This is analogous to having a cut in your skin. Initially it may hurt a little, but if it gets infected and inflamed, the pain can become unbearable.

While it's a safe bet that you're not exactly fascinated (or even clearly guided) by the above information regarding dermatomes and myotomes, the following easy-to-do self-test might help you better determine the source of your pain—if indeed you have coexistent back and leg pain. This list indicates what sort of pain or other abnormality is associated with each spinal nerve root dermatome and myotome, and then suggests a simply way to test for that abnormality:

L2 nerve root dermatome: pain or a change in sensation in the groin area. Rub your fingers symmetrically (that is, covering both sides equally) over your groin area. Do you feel numbness or an altered sensation on the leg with pain? If so, L2 may be the affected root.

L2 nerve root myotome: weakness in flexion of the hip joint or extension of the knee. To test, try a one-legged squat. Difficulty in performing the squat suggests weakness. Note: At times it can be hard to separate weakness from pain.

L3 nerve root dermatome: pain or a change in sensation in the anterior thigh to the knee. With this root, there is often knee pain. Rub your

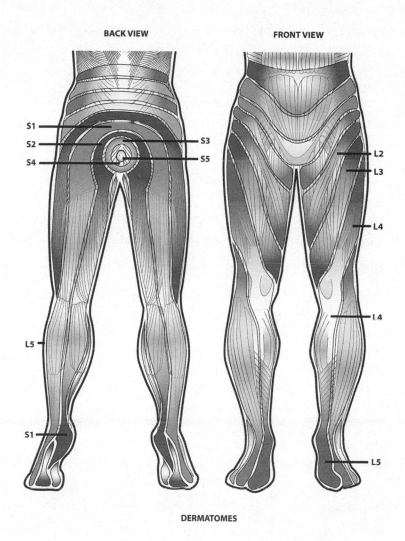

BACK VIEW   FRONT VIEW

S1
S2
S4
S3
S5

L2
L3

L4

L4

L5

S1

L5

DERMATOMES

fingers symmetrically on the front of your thighs. Do you feel numbness or an altered sensation? If so, L3 may be the affected root.

L3 nerve root myotome: weakness in flexion of the hip joint or extension of the knee. To test, try a one-legged squat. Difficulty with the squat suggests the L3 root as well.

L4 nerve root dermatome: pain or a change in sensation in the anterior thigh or along the shin. Rub your fingers symmetrically along the anterior thigh and down the shin. Do you feel numbness or an altered sensation? If so, L4 may be the affected root.

L4 nerve root myotome: weakness in the flexion of the hip joint or extension of the knee. To test, try a one-legged squat. Note: A one-legged squat highlights multiple possible connections, because the quadriceps muscle gets its nerve supply from the L2, L3, and L4 roots.

L5 nerve root dermatome: pain or a change in sensation in the lateral calf or top of the foot. Rub your fingers symmetrically along the top of your foot and onto your big toe. (If you can reach!) Do you feel numbness or a change in sensation? If so, L5 may be the affected root.

L5 nerve root myotome: weakness in the dorsiflexors of the ankle. To test, try walking on your heels. If your foot flops down, the L5 root may be the culprit.

S1 nerve root dermatome: pain or a change in sensation in the back of the calf or the bottom of the foot. Rub your fingers along the bottom of the foot toward the pinky toe. (This test is best done sitting.) Do you feel numbness or a change in sensation? If so, S1 may be the affected root.

S1 nerve root myotome: weakness in plantar flexion of the ankle. To test, walk on your toes. An inability to hold your body weight up on the toes of the painful leg may indicate that this root is the source.

The Disc Fix

If you have back pain and an MRI that shows a herniated disc, you may be offered surgery. (Don't worry; we'll talk more about the Big *S* later.) In this circumstance (back pain on its own), the surgery may or may not help. If you have back pain with leg pain and an MRI that shows the disc pushing on a nerve that matches the anatomical course of your pain syndrome, the likelihood of success with surgery will be much higher.

Herniated discs change over time. Some patients assume that once a disc has herniated, it will *stay* herniated until it's surgically repaired. This is simply not the case. Herniated discs tend to evolve in two distinct ways. First, the gel component may get smaller over time (if, for example, the water content in the gel diminishes), causing the herniation portion to shrink. This is equivalent to what happens to a grape in the sun—it shrinks and becomes a raisin. Second, the aforementioned inflammatory response can "eat away" at the disc and make it smaller.

In addition to the above factors, which singly or together may make the gel smaller, disc herniation can change due to a ligament just outside the annulus called the posterior longitudinal ligament. This ligament's job is to hold the disc away from the nerve. It has elastic properties and exerts a compressive force on any disc herniation, urging it back toward the disc space. Some disc herniations can be reduced or pushed back toward the disc space in this way. This is one of the purported mechanisms of physical therapy. Therapy takes advantage of the anterior migration of the disc that occurs when the back is in extension. (We'll explore physical therapy more in the next chapter.)

Oh, My Aching . . . Facet?

The complementary structure to the disc (which, as we saw, resides in the front of the spine) is called the facet joint (at the back of the spine). Also called the zygapophyseal joint, this paired structure (one joint on each side) may be thought of the handles of a wheelbarrow, with the wheel representing the disc space (as in the earlier illustration). These paired joints protect the disc by limiting rotation and anterior translation (one body moving forward relative to another) of the vertebral bodies. Their configuration allows for flexion—think of lifting the wheelbarrow handles off the ground. Their flexion is limited by a number of ligaments, including the so-called yellow ligament (or ligamentum flavum), which is the most elastic ligament in the body. Like so many other joints in the body, facet joints have a lining (synovium) that secretes synovial fluid, which acts as a lubricant. Also similar to other joints, the facets are vulnerable to the development of acute and chronic arthritis (arthritis being inflammation of a joint), and thus can be a source of back pain.

Facet-generated pain is more common in the older patient than the younger patient. This is likely the result of degenerative changes that affect *all* the joints in our bodies over time—the aforementioned arthritis, for example—including these facet joints of the spine.

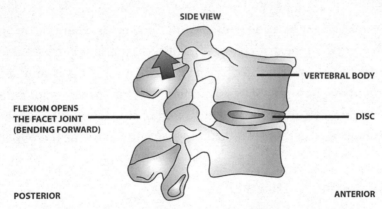

SIDE VIEW

VERTEBRAL BODY

FLEXION OPENS
THE FACET JOINT
(BENDING FORWARD)

DISC

POSTERIOR

ANTERIOR

FLEXION CAUSES THE FACET JOINTS TO OPEN AND THE DISC TO MIGRATE POSTERIORLY.

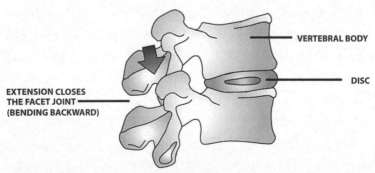

VERTEBRAL BODY

DISC

EXTENSION CLOSES
THE FACET JOINT
(BENDING BACKWARD)

EXTENSION CAUSES THE FACET JOINT TO CLOSE AND THE DISC TO MIGRATE ANTERIORLY.

As noted earlier, facet pain is more likely to be felt in the standing position. This, like the sitting pain of disc herniation, can be understood in terms of simple physics. When we stand, the joints are pushed together by gravity. If a joint is inflamed, this compression will increase the pain.

Some interesting facts (well, at least *I* think they're interesting) about the facet joints include:

- Arthritis of the facet joints results in hypertrophy (enlargement) of the bones and the ligaments. Over time, this can reduce the diameter of the spinal canal, causing the well-known and common condition of the elderly called spinal stenosis.

- The capsule of a facet joint, which is innervated similarly to the annulus of the disc, represents the mechanism of back pain in cases of facet inflammation.

- Back pain from facet joints typically arises with standing, lying prone (on the stomach), and walking, while it's relieved by lying on the side and sitting. This makes it the opposite of disc pain, which is typically worse with sitting and is relieved with standing.

- Facet joints are like any other joint in the body in a couple of ways. (1) They're lined with synovium, a thin membrane that provides lubricating synovial fluid. (2) Similar to the other joints in the body, the facet joints can be afflicted by any systemic arthritic condition, as noted above.

Diagnosing Common Types of Back Pain

Spinal Stenosis

Spinal stenosis is like prostate hypertrophy or graying of the hair—it's not a matter of *if*, but *when*. If one lives long enough, one will get it. Spinal stenosis is a favorite topic of mine because it epitomizes medicine's dichotomy of purpose: eradication of disease and promotion of health. As much as surgery would appear to be the paradigm of eradication of disease, I'll show you how, in spinal stenosis, it may be more properly conceived of as a promotion of health.

Spinal stenosis is not actually a syndrome, but an anatomic finding. Nonetheless, it's often described as if it were a syndrome. It should be understood that simply having spinal stenosis is not an issue. Many people have it and have no symptoms—and thus need no treatment. The most commonly associated syndrome is called neurogenic claudication, which means pain in the legs when you're walking.

The word *stenosis* is derived from the Greek language and means "narrowing." The narrowing of spinal stenosis is a result of the thickening of bones and ligaments in the spine. Ultimately, that thickening compromises the diameter of the canal through which the nerve roots descend when passing from the bottom of the spinal cord to exit the spinal canal and form peripheral nerves. This thickening is an example of one of the many ways in which the body's protective mechanisms end up having an unintentionally negative effect. In this case, the hypertrophic changes in the ligaments and bones of the lumbar spine, which are programmed by nature to counter wear-and-tear stresses, do so at the expense of the adjacent, traversing nerve roots. Put another way, the spine thickens with age to protect its structural integrity, and in doing so compresses the nerves that run through it.

This nerve compression can manifest as pain, numbness, heaviness of the legs, and, rarely, weakness. What makes spinal stenosis unique is that the pain typically arises only when the patient is standing or walking. Sitting or lying down typically relieves the pain. Since the patient is able to get relief by changing position, the condition can be, and often is, tolerated for a long time.

These somewhat unique features of spinal stenosis lead to an insidious restriction of many of the activities of daily living. The patient, focused on the pain, is often unaware of how much of his or her life has been altered by avoidance of this pain. Many patients never seek surgical treatment, believing that they're too old or that the gradual erosion of their repertoire of activities is a normal consequence of aging.

What patients often fail to realize, however, is that when one stops walking, two things are sure to follow: First, the body—the heart in particular—weakens from the lack of activity. Second, the brain begins to rot from a lack of variety and stimulation. By limiting walking, the patient avoids pain but loses cardiovascular fitness and brain acuity. Thus deconditioning and dementia are the unrecognized or overlooked consequences of spinal stenosis. Dementia may seem like an exaggeration, but when the brain is deprived of the stimulation and variety that being mobile provides, it can lose much of its vitality.

The effective treatment of spinal stenosis should thus be considered an empowering process—a process that promotes health, rather than a process that eliminates a disease. In fact, because spinal stenosis is a manifestation of chronic arthritis, it can never really be eliminated.

Although there are a variety of treatments employed in dealing with spinal stenosis, most of them are either ineffective or merely make the patient better temporarily. They often focus on reducing the pain rather than empowering the patient. I'm all for starting off with conservative treatments, but if the treatments employed serve only to delay the inevitable need to make room for the nerve roots surgically, the treatments may be counterproductive. For example, patients subjected to prolonged conservative treatments who ultimately opt for surgery, but only after enduring a restricted or a painful lifestyle, have the surgery in a deconditioned state, which makes recovery more difficult.

Oddly, this may be an instance where surgeons aren't aggressive enough. Often the medical doctor or family members suggest to the patient that he or she is too old for surgery. This well-meant advice may paradoxically cause the patient to have a worse result.

It never ceases to amaze me how much advice friends and family dispense when it comes to treatment of back pain. I always advise patients to respond to family or friends who have given their advice

---

Hidden Truth 14: Your Family and Friends Are Your Enemies!

---

with "What did you think of my MRI? Surely you looked at it in order to evaluate my problem. You wouldn't be so arrogant as to advise me prior to its perusal!" This usually keeps people from offering any additional "free" advice.

Roth's R$_X$: Be careful when receiving "free" advice!
Most of it ends up being overpriced! The cost of
free advice is in the perpetuation of myths.

The surgical treatment of spinal stenosis is often complicated, because it has to be individualized to each patient in terms of the level of stenosis treated, the amount of bone and ligament removed, and the need to fuse the decompressed levels. This is where dialogue between doctor and patient is essential.

Earlier, I discussed the importance of seeing a specialist early in the course of diagnosis and treatment. Spinal stenosis is a perfect example of this need. I often see patients with severe stenosis who've been treated with a variety of conservative treatments, which gave temporizing relief, or no relief at all. A sophisticated look at the MRI would have resulted in surgery as an early and appropriate treatment, based simply on the degree of stenosis and the poor expected results of other treatments.

How does spinal stenosis cause pain? To answer this question, we must look separately at how stenosis causes back versus leg pain.

- The back pain in spinal stenosis is likely the result of the arthritis of the facet joints that caused the stenosis in the first place.
- Associated multifidus muscle weakness can also cause back pain.

- The leg pain in spinal stenosis is not clearly understood. It may be a combination of the nerve roots being compressed and thus inflamed, along with the nerve roots being deprived of oxygen or blood flow from the compression.

How does spinal stenosis improve? It doesn't, on its own. The symptoms associated with the narrowing may wax and wane, particularly early on in the course of the disease. The overall trend, however, is typically to worsen slowly. Physical therapy may help temporarily. Epidural steroid injections are often helpful, particularly in the early stages, but these, too, offer only temporary relief. Most of the time, when the stenosis is severe, surgery is needed to provide more room for the traversing nerve roots.

Although *back pain* caused by spinal stenosis is often treated with surgery, the results are much less predictable than are the results for *leg pain* caused by spinal stenosis. In the setting of back pain alone, the patient is better served to pursue physical therapy and pain management.

Core Question
||||||||||||||||||||||||||||||||||||||

What Is the "Shopping Cart Sign"?

An intriguing phenomenon is so common that it's been attributed its own "sign." Some of you may find that you can "miraculously" walk longer, without pain, while in the supermarket pushing the shopping cart around. The shopping cart isn't really supplying support, in that case, but allowing you to walk with your spine in a slightly flexed position. Flexing the spine makes the spinal canal larger so that areas that are stenotic become less stenotic. The nerve roots are less compressed in this position, and thus you have less pain when walking.

Sciatica

Hidden Truth 15: Sciatica Is Not Sciatica!

In reality, this is just a semantic distinction. For years, the term *sciatica* has been indiscriminately applied to pain radiating down the leg along the course of the sciatic nerve. The name of the nerve comes from the Latin word *sciaticus,* which is derived from the Greek word *ischiadikos*—both of which are related to the hip or loin. In reality, the sciatic nerve itself is rarely the cause of pain down the leg; rather, the pain arises from lumbar roots that travel down the spinal canal and exit from the spine. These roots coalesce and, ultimately, form nerves, one of which is the sciatic nerve. A more appropriate term for this cause of pain down the leg is *radiculopathy*—inflammation of a nerve root— and not inflammation of the sciatic nerve itself.

Disc herniation is one common cause of sciatica. When a disc becomes herniated in the low back, the above-described radiculopathy can result. This is referred to as sciatica.

Another commonly diagnosed cause for sciatica (true sciatica) is a condition called the piriformis syndrome.

The Piriformis Syndrome

The piriformis muscle serves as an external rotator of the thigh and as an abductor of the hip when the leg is flexed at the hip. In cases of severe, persistent leg pain without an apparent cause shown by the lumbar MRI, imaging of the pelvis or leg is occasionally done. In rare cases, a mass is identified that truly compresses the sciatic nerve, but this is rare. The sciatic nerve actually goes right through the piriformis muscle in 20 to 33 percent of specimens, and in only a small percentage does this result in sciatica.

It's impossible to state the true incidence of the piriformis syndrome, because there's no "gold standard" for proving its diagnosis. Studies suggest that it's responsible for 6 percent of sciatica and more than half the cases of sciatica not caused by a disc herniation.[4] I think that the true percentage is far less than this. There's an effective way of disproving the diagnosis, however: Not infrequently, a patient who gets this diagnosis ends up having a discectomy and enjoying subsequent resolution of the pain.

It's a natural diagnosis to consider because, with sciatica, the pain often occurs right where the sciatic nerve penetrates the piriformis muscle. We must remember, however, that the location of a pain is not always helpful in understanding its cause.

Spondylolisthesis

This is an anatomically defined condition (a diagnosis made by an imaging study) that refers to one vertebra slipping relative to an adjacent vertebra. The term is derived from the Greek roots *spondylo* for "vertebra" and *listhesis* for "slippage." There are many causes for this condition, but the most common are labeled *degenerative* and *isthmic*.

The degenerative variety is thought to be the result of the weakening and ultimate incompetence of the facet joints. Most commonly found in women over sixty, degenerative spondylolisthesis is a consequence of the shape of the facet joints, the shape of the spine, and the weakened musculature. It occurs most commonly at the L4–5 segment of the spine.

The isthmic variety is more common in younger men and usually occurs at the L5–S1 segment. It's most commonly the result of a stress fracture of a part of the L5 bone called the pars interarticularis—an isthmus or narrowed part of the bone that connects the two larger joints above and below it. This type of stress fracture is surprisingly common. It's likely the result of an individual's spine shape, the size of the isthmus, the types of activities performed, and the growth of the patient. It occurs most often during the teenage years and may not ever be symptomatic. If it does become symptomatic, it usually does so later in life. It's often seen in gymnasts and cricket bowlers, both of whom require repetitive back extension. In the introduction, I shared with you that as a teen I experienced spondylolisthesis, but didn't know it until later when I was diagnosed with a herniated disc. The symptoms associated with this condition are typically back pain and/or leg pain. When the symptoms are severe enough to warrant treatment, it's appropriately considered a form of spinal instability.

Sacroiliac Joint Pain

Of course you remember the sacroiliac joint, the SI joint, from your favorite chapter of this book—the anatomy chapter. Well, just in case you glazed over that portion, the sacroiliac joint connects the sacrum (the bottom of the spine, just below the lumbar spine) to the ilium bones (the paired bones commonly referred to as the pelvis). It's thought to be the origin of back pain in a significant percentage of patients, but the actual percentage is debated. One of the difficulties in knowing what percentage of back pain is due to this joint is that there's no test *proving* the joint as the cause. The most reliable diagnostic test remains an injection of local anesthetic into the joint, with a subsequent resolution of the pain.

This syndrome is more commonly manifested during pregnancy, because the joint loosens during pregnancy to allow for the pelvic expansion of birth. Research using the sacroiliac anesthetic block as the diagnostic criterion suggests that nearly 20 percent of chronic low back pain may originate in this joint. The pain is felt mostly in the back and can radiate into the buttock or hip area.

Degenerative Disc Disease

This is a common anatomical finding. The vast majority of degenerative disc disease is not painful. It *may* be associated with pain, however, through several mechanisms.

First, as the height of the disc diminishes—as it does with, for example, age—the ligamentous structures that provide support lose their tension. This allows for potential "toggling" between the adjacent vertebral bodies. Although this toggling is virtually never identifiable on dynamic (flexion/extension) X-rays, it's suggested by some surgeons to cause a slight amount of instability—instability not detectable radiographically, but inferred clinically because of the pain. This inferred instability is then used to justify a fusion procedure. You'll learn in chapter 7 that this is probably the most common rationale for surgery, despite being unsubstantiated by the body of available literature.

Another etiology for back pain connected to degenerative disc disease is the transference of stress from the disc space to the facet joints with the loss of height of the disc space, and subsequent pain related to this increased stress.

Spinal Instability

Often the most difficult of back conditions to diagnose, and certainly the most controversial, spinal instability assumes an excess of motion between two spinal segments that results in pain or compromised function. The controversy in diagnosis arises because, in the majority of cases, the motion is not demonstrated, but only inferred (by the presence of pain). We know that pain can be the result of excess motion. Since there *is* pain, we infer motion. The problem is that pain is often due to other factors, so inferring that a given pain is due to undetectable motion is a stretch. Surgery based on such an inference has a poorer success rate than surgery done in cases of demonstrable instability. In my opinion, this circular logic (and the subsequent surgical treatments that follow) is the main reason that spine surgery has developed such a poor reputation.

While instability *sometimes* has to be inferred (the controversial cases), it's often obvious on an X-ray. I had a patient who'd had terrible back pain for a number of years. The pain would come on with activity and was relieved when he rested in bed. The patient had tried physical therapy many times and found that the therapy just made the pain worse. When I saw the patient in my office, the physical exam was unremarkable, as was the MRI. Because the history of the pain was so "mechanical" in nature, I obtained standing flexion and extension X-rays, which showed a clear motion between the L4 and L5 vertebral bodies: L4 moved forward relative to L5 when the patient flexed forward. (The MRI didn't reveal the laxity between the two vertebrae because the pictures were "static"—done with the patient lying down and immobile.) Having seen clear evidence of instability, I treated the patient by fusing the L4 body to the L5 body, which resulted in much less pain.

Most of the time, however, such dynamic instability is not evident and the diagnosis is made on inference. For example, the facet joints may display excess water content, suggesting stress on them from instability; or the marrow of a vertebra may show edema, suggesting excess stress on the bone from instability. Spondylolisthesis, discussed earlier, is a condition in which the alignment of the vertebral bodies is altered, also suggesting instability.

How does instability cause pain? Presumably, the supporting structures are stressed by the movement caused by the loosened attachment between any two vertebral bones. This movement results in pain. Instability improves when motion is diminished. This diminishment can happen over time. For example, ligaments may shorten or become scarred and stiffen, decreasing motion; likewise, muscle strengthening may reduce the motion across the abnormal segment by increasing tone. Finally, surgery eliminates the motion if the two bones are fused together. (We'll discuss fusion in chapter 7.)

Am I Just Too Fat?

Hidden Truth 16: Weight Loss Does Not Improve Back Pain!

Patients are often told that their back pain will disappear if they lose weight. This theory seems to make sense. Compression of the disc spaces must be proportional to a person's body weight, and simple physics would dictate that bending forward with more weight results in increased leverage on the lower back. The reality, however, is that when excess weight is looked at as an independent contributor to back pain, the results are not convincing. Put another way, if the weight could be magically removed instantly, back pain wouldn't predictably be improved.[5]

Does this mean that overweight people with back pain shouldn't try to lose weight? Of course not, but they should focus on the process of weight loss rather than on the number of pounds lost. If one looks at the strategy of patients who *successfully* lose weight, it's usually a combination of both less caloric intake (or a different type of caloric intake) and an increased caloric expenditure. This caloric expenditure can be achieved by aerobic exercise or muscle strengthening. In my experience, it's the exercise component of the weight loss (and mostly the muscle strengthening) that brings about the control of back pain—not the pounds lost. Put another way, if a patient sets out to lose weight to aid in his or her back pain by eating less and exercising more, there will almost always be a reduction in back pain even if there's no weight loss. If the attempt to lose weight is handled only with a change in diet, however, the success rate is lower.

Roth's R$_x$: If you're overweight and have back pain, focus on the exercise portion of your weight loss program. Even if you don't lose weight, it's a safe bet that your back will improve.

While I've had fun mocking the status quo of diagnosis, I do have compassion for people who can't seem to get a handle on their pain. With those folks especially in mind, I'll turn now to the more traditional ways people can manage their pain. Early in this book, I quoted Maslow—"If your only tool is a hammer, you tend to see every problem as a nail"—to illustrate the idea that choosing one type of practitioner will result in one type of treatment. In the next chapter, I'll teach you about the various options out there, in case you want to trade in that hammer for a wrench—or readjust the tool belt altogether by means other than by the Hidden Core Workout.

The Gist

- I don't expect you to diagnose yourself, but an understanding of the disc and facet joints, and of common conditions of the back, will enhance your communication with your healthcare provider.

CHAPTER 6

THE NONSURGICAL TREATMENT OF BACK PAIN

PATIENTS face a confusing array of choices for the treatment of pain. You've already learned that where you start and who you work with, rather than the nature of the pain itself, often defines the treatment that you get. This chapter provides an overview of nonsurgical treatments available. Understanding the rationale for these treatments will help you make decisions for treatment of your back pain.

Hidden Truth 17: Too Many Choices Can Be Worse Than Not Enough Choices!

When it comes to choices, the more the better, right? Not necessarily. In fact, too many choices can be paralyzing. Ever go to Disney World and see all the "lands" to visit . . . and find yourself unable to decide where to start? How do you know where to begin the journey? Well, it's not so different when a patient with back pain considers the staggering number of treatment options.

It turns out that human beings have a difficult time with too much information. A landmark study looked at the correlation between the number of options and the ease of choice. In the study, shoppers were given the option to taste and potentially purchase jam in a supermarket. One group was presented six flavor options, while another group was presented twenty-four. It turns out that while more shoppers visited the area where there were more options, more shoppers actually bought jam in the environment of fewer options. This study suggests that we're attracted to having many options, but too many options can make deciding harder. The end result might be no result at all.[1]

USE YOUR INSTINCT

We all have instinct, though most of us underrate and distrust it. Our instinct is an inborn sense of what we need and what we should avoid. A baby can suck milk, for example, without any instruction; the action is instinctual. With time, though, each individual's inborn instinct evolves into a well-developed system of thought that's individualized to each of us based on our own experiences and makeup.

I believe that human instinct develops and becomes more complex in a similar fashion to the visual system. In the case of the visual system, we go from the rudimentary ability to recognize simple lines and shapes to recognizing something as complex as our grandmother's face in profile, and we do this effortlessly. This development, which requires time, is the result of a tremendous networking of neurons that coalesce and connect with each other effortlessly as we simply *use* our eyes.

A similar phenomenon occurs with the development of instinct, whereby our decision-making system becomes more sophisticated and functional over time. Again, this happens to each of us simply by *living*. This acquired instinct enables us to trust or not trust another person after a brief encounter. Likewise, it enables us to accept or reject a proposed treatment for back pain after initial consideration, and to analyze whether an ongoing treatment is worthwhile. Instinct isn't capricious or arbitrary; it's extremely sophisticated and, more importantly, individualized to each person.

Roth's R$_X$: Understand and accept that there's often no "correct" choice. Trust your instincts and be prepared to change directions if needed.

PAIN MANAGEMENT

A new field in medicine, pain management, has recently emerged. Though relatively new on the scene, this discipline has quickly become established in nearly all communities and academic centers. Pain management, as its name would suggest, tends to prioritize the reduction of pain. This differs from surgery, which not only reduces the pain (or so the patient and surgeon hope), but aims to fix it.

The field of pain management draws from the fields of anesthesia, physiatry (physical medicine and rehabilitation), and neurology. The field's quick ascent as a distinct discipline reflects, in part, the difficulty that pain presents to the healthcare provider. Patients in pain require time and energy. Once considered a "dumping ground" for these difficult patients, the field of pain management developed quickly as a safe and efficient way for overworked and overwhelmed practitioners to dispense medications to patients on a routine basis.

To understand pain management, you must have an overview of what's in the practitioner's repertoire to help you with pain.

Medications

Many different types of medicines are used to treat pain. The following is a general overview. As you read through this menu, bear in mind that *all* medications are a double-edged sword: With every benefit there's a downside as well. Medications work best when given for a specific purpose and for a limited time, limiting the potential for downside effects.

Nonsteroidal Anti-Inflammatories

As their name implies, anti-inflammatories are medications that reduce inflammation. There are two types: nonsteroidal anti-inflammatory drugs, or NSAIDs, and steroidals (see below). NSAIDs are variants of aspirin, the prototypical anti-inflammatory. These are the most commonly used medications for pain, and usually the most effective.

The side effects of NSAIDs include the inhibition of platelets, and thus they have the potential to cause bleeding. They can also cause irritation of the gastrointestinal tract as well as kidney toxicity, even when given in recommended doses. They're used as pain relievers and to treat inflammatory conditions, including arthritis—basically any condition that ends in "itis" (meaning "inflammation of"), such as appendicitis.

Steroidal Anti-Inflammatories

Steroids are also anti-inflammatory medications, but they work by a slightly different mechanism than the NSAIDs. They're stronger than nonsteroidal anti-inflammatories and should be used cautiously. They can cause retention of fluid and salt, as well as cognitive and emotional changes. They're more toxic than NSAIDs when used over a long term. Furthermore, they can cause the adrenal gland to stop producing its own steroids, which it does as a reaction to stress. If the body can no longer produce its own steroids, it may be left vulnerable in times of stress. Steroids are given orally or intravenously for inflammatory conditions, often when nonsteroidals don't suffice.

Narcotics

Narcotics are tightly controlled in the United States by the Drug Enforcement Administration because of their propensity for abuse. (They're highly addictive.) These drugs control pain by a different mechanism than anti-inflammatories. Rather than diminishing the pain-causing inflammation, narcotics simply reduce the pain. In addition, they create euphoria, help with sleep, and cause constipation. All narcotics lose their efficacy over time. Continued use changes a patient's tolerance for pain.

Hidden Truth 18: Pain Medication Causes More Pain!

The treatment of back pain with narcotics has a long and controversial history. Recent reviews of the literature fail to show a clear benefit from this type of treatment. Furthermore, narcotics can lead to potential complications. In my practice, I often see a clash between the approach of certain pain management doctors and my own. Philosophically, there are two camps: The first believes that pain should be treated aggressively and early with pain medication so as to avoid the development of pathological alternative responses, such as avoiding activity. The other camp (which I'm in) believes that pain medication, in the long run, creates more pain. In the *short* term, however, pain medication is often necessary and helpful, as it allows for activity.

There's much scientific support for the camp I belong to.[2] Have you ever wondered why narcotics work in the first place? And why we "happen" to have receptors in our body for narcotics? The answer to this mystery is that we have endogenous (natural) opiates that circulate all the time through our bloodstream, providing natural control of pain. These circulating narcotics are called endorphins. When we introduce pain medication into our bloodstream, we disrupt the body's natural balance between endorphins and receptors for the endorphins.

When pain medication is taken over a long period of time, the body thinks that there's too much of its natural painkiller, and it responds by reducing the number of *receptors* for the endorphins, to restore balance. What happens is that the balance is reset to a state where there are more endorphins binding to fewer receptors. When the pain medication is stopped or wears off, the body finds itself with too few receptors. As a result, the pain threshold is lowered and the patient is actually more susceptible to pain.

In addition, there's recent evidence that the chronic use of narcotics directly alters—indeed, eases—the transmission of pain in the spinal cord. In other words, narcotics, over time, make it easier for pain to go through the synapses in the spinal cord and reach the brain.

Roth's R$_X$: Decide which camp you're in. If you want to go with pain medication, consider the possibility that it not only won't help, but may hurt!

Analgesics

Analgesics are typically injected or applied topically—that is, directly to the skin. They're more effective when injected, but this isn't a practical way of taking them on a routine basis. The topical administration is limited in how much the drug penetrates the skin. The most common application is with the Lidoderm patch. This patch is applied on the affected skin and releases lidocaine, which numbs the skin and the area just beneath. Because of analgesics' short-lived efficacy, they're more often used for diagnostic purposes than for therapeutic purposes.

Muscle Relaxants

Muscle relaxants are prescribed to address the secondary muscle spasm that can accompany pain. They help minimize the anxiety that sometimes comes along with (and can exacerbate or amplify) pain. They also help a person sleep. Like narcotics, they're potentially addictive and should be administered and used with caution.

Antidepressants

Antidepressants work by increasing the amount of norepinephrine or serotonin in the synapses of nerves. These targeted substances are neurotransmitters, meaning that they help mediate the communication between nerves in the brain. Antidepressants have a subtler and less predictable effect on pain than the previous types of drugs discussed, and typically the onset of relief is delayed, often by as long as a few days. Antidepressants are used for leg pain more than back pain, or for back pain when there's a superimposed element of depression. In general, the efficacy of antidepressants is much less predictable than that of the aforementioned medications.

Antiseizure Medications

Antiseizure medications are being used with increasing frequency for pain. Originally used for seizure disorders only, they stabilize nerve cell membranes and make the nerves less "excitable." In my experience, their effect, as with antidepressants, is difficult to predict. They're most effective for neuropathy (pain or numbness arising from a diseased nerve) and less effective in spine-derived pain.

Injections

There are a variety of types of injections used by pain management doctors. Injections have the advantage of allowing for a greater concentration of a drug in a specific area. Furthermore, their onset of action is usually faster than that of oral or topical medications. Injections also allow for the use of certain drugs that can't be ingested.

Epidural Injection

This is the administration of a liquid steroid into the space just outside the dura, the tough membrane covering the nerves within the spinal canal. An epidural injection is most effective when administered under the guidance of a fluoroscope (an X-ray machine that shows the tip of the needle just before injection). Most pain management doctors won't administer an epidural injection more than three times in a six-month period due to steroidal toxicity.

Facet Injection

This is the administration of either a steroid or an analgesic (or both) to a facet joint. The injection can be into the joint itself (called an intra-articular injection) or into the vicinity of the nerve that innervates the joint (a medial branch block). These injections can be either therapeutic or diagnostic.

Selective Root Block

This is a certain type of epidural injection. A selective root block requires a smaller amount of anesthetic, and the purpose of the injection is *only* diagnostic. This block is to determine whether a specific nerve is what's causing the pain in an individual patient.

Sympathetic Ganglion Block

In this injection, a needle, under the guidance of a fluoroscope, is passed into the vicinity of what's known as a sympathetic ganglion found in the thoracic spine. The sympathetic ganglia are part of the body's "sympathetic system," an accessory system of nerves that, among other things, helps regulate temperature and vasodilatation (widening of the blood vessels). This injection is typically used either for a syndrome called reflex sympathetic dystrophy or for a syndrome of excessive sweating.

Discogram Injection

Performed by a surgeon or a radiologist, a discogram—which involves a diagnostic injection—is a controversial test sometimes used to determine whether a specific disc is the cause of a patient's pain. The idea is to place a needle into one or more disc spaces and then inject the disc with saline. The patient, who ideally doesn't know which disc has been injected, then says whether the injection was painful and whether the pain was similar to the pain that he or she has been trying to make better.

This treatment is controversial, because it's not clear that the results are reproducible. In addition, discograms produce many false positives, suggesting that a disc is painful when it's actually not, and false negatives, suggesting that a disc is *not* painful when it actually is.

The test is also sometimes abused, in that it's used as a rationale for further treatment. Often the person giving the test is the one who stands to profit by any subsequent procedures. This introduces unavoidable bias.

Invasive Pain Management Procedures

Finally, there are certain invasive procedures done in pain management. These procedures are philosophically different from the procedures done by a traditional surgeon. Surgeons typically theorize a cause for the pain and then seek to rectify the problem via a surgical procedure. Pain management specialists, on the other hand, have a range of invasive procedures that don't (necessarily) suppose a cause: These are utilized simply to *treat* pain.

Dorsal Column Stimulation

Dorsal column stimulation uses an electrode placed over the dorsal (rear) surface of the spinal cord, causing an ensuing vibration in an area that feels painful to the patient. As noted earlier, this stimulator utilizes the gate theory of pain: A reflexive diminution of pain transmission is created by a surplus of vibration sensation over the same area of skin (dermatome) in which the pain is felt. This entire stimulator unit is implanted under the skin and doesn't have to be removed. The control panel can be programmed by the patient through the skin, with a magnet. Trial and error is often called for on the part of the patient to arrive at the optimal setting.

Intrathecal Delivery

The intrathecal pump, also implanted, delivers medicine (usually morphine) into the spinal fluid that bathes the nerves. Morphine helps with pain and lets the patient avoid the side effects of oral narcotics, such as lethargy and constipation. The pump's use is limited to some extent by the patient's tolerance for the drug, as is the case with other narcotic delivery methods. It delivers the narcotic at a programmable rate, which can be adjusted by the patient to control the pain.

Percutaneous Discectomy

This is a procedure performed by both surgeons and, more recently, pain management doctors. Although there are variations of this procedure, it most commonly involves the placement of a tube into the disc space through the skin under X-ray guidance, and the subsequent removal of the nucleus pulposus.

It's less invasive than the typical microdiscectomy (discectomy done under magnification—more on this in the next chapter), but also inferior. Typically, removal of disc material from within the disc space is done with the hope that it will allow the herniated portion, which can't itself be safely extracted, to move away from the compressed nerve. One interesting fact that I always come back to when judging this procedure was discovered by a study done several decades ago. At that time a similar percutaneous procedure was used to inject a substance called chymopapain into the disc space to "dissolve" the disc material. This study found that the procedure had merit, helping about 75 percent of the patients. However, it also compared the technique to a placebo, in which a needle was put into the disc space but none of the agent was injected—and in the placebo group, nearly half of the patients experienced significant relief! This suggests that *any* spinal procedure will potentially help 50 percent of the patients by the placebo effect alone.[3] The results that I see coming out of the literature for the percutaneous discectomy aren't much better than the established placebo effect.

A percutaneous discectomy allows for a slightly smaller incision than does the traditional microdiscectomy; however, it also substitutes an endoscope for a microscope, which means substituting 2-D vision for 3-D vision. This overall trade-off makes the percutaneous discectomy an inferior procedure, in my opinion. In the next chapter, on surgery, I'll discuss why you shouldn't always be persuaded by the term "minimally invasive," because of just such a lack of efficacy.

Kyphoplasty

Kyphoplasty is a treatment used mostly in cases of a compression fracture of a vertebral body, such as can occur with osteoporosis. The treatment is typically done within eight weeks of the onset of symptoms. The most common symptom is back pain that worsens when someone is sitting or standing. An MRI is often done to determine whether the fracture is acute or subacute, and whether the fracture happened recently. This latter is important, because while computed tomography (CT) scans and plain X-rays can show a fracture, only an MRI can show whether the fracture is relatively new. (Kyphoplasty is not effective on an old fracture.)

Kyphoplasty is a minimally invasive procedure that's done with fluoroscopic guidance. A needle is inserted into the fractured vertebral body. A balloon is then inflated through the needle, creating a cavity in the fractured bone that accommodates the introduction of a type of cement. This cement, injected still under fluoroscopic guidance, supplies strength and support to the vertebral body. The expectation is that there will be less pain with the bearing of weight.

Hands-On Therapies

I was plagued with plantar fasciitis several years ago and began to think that it would never get better. After eight months of no progress, a friend of mine who practices physical therapy suggested that I try therapy for my pain—specifically, longitudinal massage to "break down" the scar tissue and to "train" it to align properly as it healed. I was skeptical, to say the least, but I gave it a try because nothing else had worked.

Not only did it work, it literally cured me after a couple of treatments. It was my first experience with connective tissue modeling; in addition, it was an introduction to the concept of scar tissue as "live" tissue, with the ability to adapt and strengthen when properly stressed.

My practice, like that of a physical therapist, takes advantage of the adaptability of connective tissues. This, too, is based on the body's inherent ability to strengthen when properly stressed.

Another friend of mine is a chiropractor. He has treated me numerous times. I often test his "hands" by asking him to evaluate my back without giving him with any information as to where I hurt. It never ceases to amaze me how quickly he identifies the spastic muscle, say, and how effective the techniques applied to the muscle are in reducing pain. The point with both these examples is that a practitioner's hands can be trained to become effective tools in the treatment of soft-tissue pain.

There's a definite art to hands-on therapies for pain arising from connective and muscle soft tissue. This is a difficult area to navigate, however, as there are so many specialists (including chiropractors, osteopaths, and physical therapists, for instance) and so many different techniques (such as Rolfing and active release therapy). There's no perfect way to determine which specialty or technique is best suited for your specific needs. Once you've selected a specialty, there's similarly no perfect way to select among providers, short of a recommendation followed by trial and error. Finally, depending on the circumstances, the cost for such services may or may not be paid for by your insurance company.

The other limitation in treating the muscles and connective tissues is in knowing whether these sore tissues are the *primary* source of your pain or an *epiphenomenon* of your pain. When patients come to me with back pain, they often have areas of muscle spasm that are contributing to their pain. These areas of muscle spasm are often not the primary pathology, however, and thus treatments may yield only temporary benefits. Treating muscle spasm that occurs secondarily to a herniated disc is analogous to patching your ceiling when there's a leak in the roof.

> ## Core Concept
> |||||||||||||||||||||||||||||||||||||||||
>
> There's increasing interest in the role of circulating hormones as media-
> tors or catalysts for many of the actions of individual cells. For example,
> in the world of dieting, the old calorie in–calorie out concept of weight
> loss has been modified to take into account the underlying hormonal
> environment. In the case of dieting, insulin levels may play a significant
> role in how those incoming calories are handled by the body.
>
> Likewise, the hormone oxytocin is now viewed as a mediator that
> calms and connects. In contrast to epinephrine, which allows for a "fight
> or flight" response, oxytocin allows for healing. It's also been shown to
> help the brain "undo" its connections and thus be open to the formation
> of new connections. This accounts for oxytocin's role in the formation of
> new relationships and love interests. Exercise is thought to act in a way
> similar to oxytocin and may actually cause the direct release of oxytocin.
>
> Massage therapy, as well as other hands-on therapies, has been
> shown to release oxytocin. Interestingly, infants who are simply touched
> more tend to gain more weight than those touched less.[4]

You may find yourself paying out of pocket for what turn out to be only temporary periods of reprieve. That gets old (and expensive) fast. The other limitation of these treatments is that they put you in a passive position—you become dependent on the therapist to treat your pain.

Muscle and Connective Tissue Therapies

Therapy on the muscles and connective tissues comes in many forms, including Rolfing, structural integration, Hellerwork, neuromuscular therapy, myofascial release, and active release techniques. These ther apies are done by therapists trained in each particular technique. The training varies in terms of rigor and consistency. Although the varia- tions and distinctions among this group are significant, it is beyond the scope of this book to detail them. It's clear, however, that such hands-on therapy can be helpful in back pain.[5]

Muscle and connective tissue manipulation as a pain management option is most likely to be successful if muscle or fascia is the primary cause of pain. Muscles can cause pain when injured, of course, but also when not used. In the latter case, the pain may arise from an ensuing stiffness, from an alteration of the closely related function of the joints, or from a change in posture or form.

To understand how and why such treatments are effective, we need to know a bit more about musculature. Striated muscle, which is the type responsible for voluntary movement of body parts, is tissue that can contract (shorten its length) and thereby apply a force across a joint. That force can result in either motion or stabilization. Muscle tissue receives a rich blood supply and has a rich nerve innervation, the latter providing the brain feedback on the relative contraction and force (stress and strain) that a muscle is applying at any given time. In addition, there's a rich network of pain fibers in the connective tissue that surrounds each muscle. These pain fibers explain muscles' capacity to cause pain.

A muscle contracts by causing individual muscle filaments to slide together, creating force. When a muscle is passively stretched, it can also generate a *counter*force that comes from the connective tissue sheaths around the muscle fibers. When a muscle contracts at the same time it's being stretched, the forces are highest, as both of these factors contribute. This has a particular significance in the mechanics of the spine, because when you quickly bend forward, tremendous force is created in your back muscles.

Throughout this book I've emphasized the spine's capacity to adapt. The muscles that line the spine and stabilize the spine are the most adaptive structures in the spinal column. They can change shape and acquire strength over a period of weeks. This is in contrast to the discs, which are also adaptive, but at a much slower rate. The various structures of the spinal column react to stress in one of two ways. If there's

In addition to these benefits from muscle pressure, the application of pressure to connective tissue can alter the electrical environment of the intracellular and extracellular spaces within that tissue—a process that aligns the collagen fibrils (important constituents of connective tissue), promotes growth of capillaries, and encourages the synthesis of collagen. Put simply, this type of therapy makes the tissue stronger and healthier and can modify scar tissue as well as structural tissue. Collagen fibers (made up of fibrils) connect to each other with hydrogen bonds, and when external pressure is applied, those bonds become more aligned and stronger. This, too, strengthens the connective tissue. Exercise aids manual therapy with this strengthening.

Connective tissue that surrounds and permeates muscles is actually heated by hands-on therapies such as Rolfing. Through a process called thixotropy, the connective tissue then becomes more like a liquid and less like a gel. This allows for a reorientation of the connective tissue, which results in improved flexibility and strength and decreased pain.

Acupuncture

Acupuncture is frequently requested by patients as a noninvasive treatment for back pain. Despite targeted research, Western medicine has yet to come up with a complete and substantiated explanation for the positive effects that acupuncture often delivers. Developed in China, acupuncture alleviates an inharmonious balance between the extremes (yin and yang) of the life force (qi).

Over the last twenty years I've seen some patients' back pain respond favorably to this treatment, though I've been unable to predict who these patients would be. More importantly, such improvements have nearly always been temporary; and because the cost is often not covered by insurance, the out-of-pocket burden can be prohibitive. Nonetheless, acupuncture is a safe and a viable option for the patient with the patience to try alternative treatments that may not be permanent and with the financial means to pay for them.

too much stress, they'll fatigue and sustain injury. Whe
applied correctly, however, they'll adapt by strengthenin,
this sweet spot earlier.

Muscles hypertrophy (become larger and stronger) in i
exercise. This hypertrophy can come about in two ways. F
trained for endurance, the muscles increase their capacity fo
function with a higher density of mitochondria and vascula.
which allows for better delivery of oxygen and better energy proc
When muscles are trained for power, the actual *fibers* hypert
When you work the hidden core, you're training the muscles foi
endurance and power.

On the flip side, muscle inactivity leads to the loss of muscle m
Not only does the muscle become thinner, but it also shortens a
becomes stiffer.[6] As a consequence, any joint that a diminished musc
serves also loses mobility.

This relationship between the muscles and the joints is an example
of the symbiotic relationship that exists among all of the participating
structures and systems of the body. Although any explanation of pain
sources invariably lists the structures/systems separately, it's obvious
that there's a complicated dynamic connecting any dysfunction to the
other related structures.

Likewise, therapies have benefits that cross structure/system bound-
aries. Manual or other variants of applying pressure to muscles have
been shown to have the following beneficial effects:

- Pain relief
- Immune system boosting
- Vasodilatation from local chemical activation (more blood supply)
- Recruitment of blood supply to the muscles
- Reduction of muscle spasm
- Facilitation of healing
- Stimulation of local metabolism
- Increased lymphatic drainage (decreased swelling)

Recent studies have demonstrated a consistent short-term benefit for back pain from acupuncture. However, it's difficult to separate this effect from the placebo effect.[7]

McKenzie Physical Therapy

Developed by Robin McKenzie, a physical therapist from New Zealand, this type of physical therapy underscores the revelation that the nucleus pulposus (gel in the center of the disc) moves posteriorly toward the nerve roots when the spine is flexed (with bending or sitting), while it moves anteriorly when the spine is extended (with lying down or lying on the belly with the upper back elevated). As you may recall, the facet joints behave in the opposite manner, becoming compressed with the patient standing and "unloaded," and decompressed with the patient sitting.

This therapy is most successfully applied by McKenzie-trained physical therapists on patients with herniated discs that cause pain with sitting. The patient is placed into a position of extension repeatedly during the day to help move the nucleus pulposus anteriorly and simultaneously to take pressure off the nerve root, allowing the annulus to heal. This is the one type of therapy I know of that actually seeks to move a herniated disc back into position.

As an essential first step, the clinician needs to look at the patient's MRI and judge whether McKenzie physical therapy is likely to work. In my practice, I've seen multiple instances of a patient having been put through McKenzie physical therapy for weeks without benefit, when the MRI could have showed at the outset—had the clinician correctly read it—that it was very unlikely to work. In my opinion, any healthcare provider who recommends the therapy should first order and review an MRI. For example, if the disc isn't fully herniated through the annulus, McKenzie physical therapy is ideal. If the disc is fully extruded, however, it's less likely to work. If the decision for therapy is based only on the radiologist's general report of a herniated disc, this will lead to a physical therapy that isn't ideally matched to the patient's specific disc herniation.

Lumbar Traction

VAX-D (for vertebral axial decompression) is a well-known brand of lumbar traction machine often presented as an option to patients with a herniated disc. The decompression process elongates the spine with a machine. In certain ways, it's conceptually similar to the aforementioned McKenzie method. By applying traction to the back, the machine creates a negative pressure in the disc space and facilitates a reduction of nucleus pulposus back into the disc space. In addition, the posterior longitudinal ligament is stretched, which helps pull the disc away from the nerve.

Here, too, the preoperative MRI should always be reviewed in the context of potential traction therapy as a predictor of success. Not all anatomic disc herniations should be subjected to this treatment. Just as is the case with McKenzie physical therapy, a disc bulge, as opposed to an extruded disc, is the type of herniation most likely to respond to traction treatment.

The literature looking at efficacy for various forms of lumbar traction has been modest, particularly when treatment is compared to the natural history of the symptoms from a disc herniation. It's hard to prove that doing the traction is better than doing nothing. Though I've seen remarkable successes, I do think this therapy should be applied carefully. Overall, it's expensive and time-consuming, but not dangerous. It represents one of many therapies that are typically utilized early in the course of disc herniation, during which time there's typically a favorable natural history that could make such treatment an unnecessary expense. (Remember that most cases of acute back pain improve naturally.)

Mattress "Therapy"

Believe it or not, while there are myriad types of pain management therapy, the lowly mattress may play an important role in mitigating your pain—and also may be your worst enemy. Since one-third of your life is spent in bed, miserable nights filled with back pain should be addressed, despite the lack of science available to guide us.

I've spent years trying to understand and organize the science of mattress selection for my patients. Theoretically, those who suffer from a herniated disc should benefit from, and prefer, a hard mattress, while those with spinal stenosis should opt for a softer mattress that allows for more settling. This is explained by the same forces that McKenzie physical therapy and traction utilize: When the mattress is hard, the back assumes an extended position, while a softer mattress allows for slightly more flexion. The kind of mattress a person would most benefit from is very difficult to predict, however, due to the general difficulty of comparing mattresses over a period of time. How many people have two beds in their house and can really compare them?

Many patients are disappointed after purchasing a new mattress to help with their back pain. This seems to reflect more the general inability of any particular mattress to predictably make a difference than an error in deciding which type of mattress to buy. In the end, I've decided that the approach should be practical. If the current mattress suffices, the mattress is a keeper. If the mattress makes for miserable nights, however, either start with a firm mattress with a soft "pillow top"—or, if you already have a firm mattress, switch to a soft one.

Studies that assess behavioral therapy in promoting sleep show that it does help with sleep and is also modestly helpful with chronic pain. This underscores the potential benefit of a comfortable mattress.[8] The behavioral techniques that are used in sleep therapy include having patients leave the bedroom if sleep doesn't come within fifteen minutes, engage in nonstimulating activity, and then return to the bedroom to try again. This therapy also tries to disabuse patients of their unrealistic ideas of the danger of sleep deprivation. (Sound familiar?) Finally, patients are given relaxation techniques that include deep breathing, muscle relaxation, and autogenic training and imaging (using images that promote relaxation).

Roth's R_X: Don't underestimate the power of a comfy
mattress and sound sleep. Chronic pain leads to
poor sleep, and poor sleep can increase pain.

Osteoporosis

Prevention and Cure

Osteoporosis is a disease that highlights our need for preventive medicine. We know much about osteoporosis, thanks to research as well as to technology such as bone density exams. We also know the demographics that are most likely affected by osteoporosis and the micronutrient sufficiency that can prevent or control it. I see many cases of weakened spines due to osteoporosis. My prescription is always exercise.

Osteoporosis, which is characterized by loss of bone density, is a condition more commonly found in women than men. The condition progresses silently over a number of years and often becomes recognized only when the patient suffers a fracture of one of the weakened bones anywhere in the body.

In the spine, the disease is often discovered after a compression fracture occurs—that is, the "flattening" or "wedging" of a bone. Such a fracture typically comes on suddenly and, in someone with osteoporosis, may be the result of a trivial trauma such as sitting down on a chair. The pain can be intense and is felt when one is standing and relieved when one is lying down (other than when turning in bed).

If a patient has experienced several of these fractures, he or she may develop kyphosis—a forward bending of the spine. This is one cause of the loss of height that occurs with aging. A spine that curves forward causes the back muscles to work overtime trying to restore balance, which can cause back pain or back fatigue.

The two major protections against osteoporosis are exercise and hormones (estrogen in women and testosterone in men). The best exercises are weight-bearing exercises like the ones in the Hidden Core Workout! Running is a better stimulant for bone production than walking, while walking is better than swimming. (Swimming's one weakness is that it isn't particularly protective against osteoporosis.) After starting a program of exercise, most patients who are at risk for osteoporosis should start on a vitamin D supplement and consider a calcium supplement as well. Vitamin D absorption can also be achieved through daily exposure to the sun.

Lifestyle adaptations that can be helpful in preventing osteoporosis include quitting smoking and lowering alcohol consumption. Additionally, a number of medications have been successful in the treatment of osteoporosis. The most common class of medications prescribed is bisphosphonates, which slow bone loss by blocking the osteoclasts, the bone cells that remove bone. Other medication options include estrogen supplements (or estrogen receptor modulators), human parathyroid hormone, and prescription-strength vitamin D.

Hot Versus Cold Compresses

"Which is better? Hot compresses or cold?" If only I had a buck for every time a patient asked me that! I always answer the question with a disappointing "It depends."

Ice works by diverting blood supply and thus diminishing inflammation. It also slows the speed of nerve conduction, which can in turn reduce spasm of the muscles. Ice can also numb tissues, directly reducing pain in that way.

Heat, on the other hand, serves a more reparative role. It increases blood supply and thus increases inflammation and facilitates tissue repair. One *might* surmise that early on in the course of pain, ice would be favored, while later in the course, heat would be the choice. My experience has been that theory is a poorer predictor of success than is trial and error. I would advise you to try both ice and heat—but start with ice if the pain has been present less than seventy-two hours and with heat if the pain has been present more than seventy-two hours.

And don't set your heart on either modality, because neither is likely to make a huge difference.[9]

Roth's R$_X$: When it comes to the application of heat and cold, theory is a poorer predictor of success than trial and error.

Integrative Therapies

In the last decade or so, the word *integrative* has replaced the word *alternative* in the terms "alternative medicine" and "alternative therapies," and with good reason. The word *alternative* used to carry a stigma, an implication that methods not based on traditional medicine or medical practice were somehow rooted in tomfoolery and "woo-woo" magical thinking. But more and more, homeopathy and alternative healing have been accepted and studied widely in the world of traditional science, to the point that some medical schools have added integrative medicine as a field of study. Below, are a few integrative treatments or therapies for pain relief that I feel are worthy of mention.

Prolotherapy
The integrative practice of prolotherapy is so named because the treatment proliferates (grows) new ligament tissue in areas where it has

> ## Core Question
> |||||||||||||||||||||||||||||||||||||
>
> *What Is Chiropractic?*
>
> From the Greek *kheiro* and *praktikos*, meaning "done by hand," the field of chiropractic traces its origins to the nineteenth century and a practitioner in Iowa named Daniel David Palmer. It has had a history of emphasizing the relationship between structure and function. From its inception, it has distinguished itself from orthodox medicine by espousing the restoration of health rather than the eradication of disease. Chiropractic uses spinal manipulation and adjustments in conjunction with the body's natural healing capacity to effect change.
>
> Chiropractic became alienated from orthodox medicine in part due to litigation with the American Medical Association that went on for more than fifty years. This history of litigation and some "extremist" practices within the field have tarnished chiropractic's reputation and obscured its philosophical and holistic underlying tenets. Chiropractic should be considered separately from these tarnishing factors.

become weak. (*Prolo* is short for *proliferation*.) Prolotherapy involves the use of an injectable agent of dextrose, or sugar water, into the spine. Dextrose is thought to trigger the body's natural inflammatory response, which grows scar tissue and causes subsequent stiffening of the supporting structures, thereby helping heal the weakened structures.

Balneotherapy

This therapy, derived from the Latin word for "bath," involves soaking the body in water supplemented with minerals such as sulfur. It has been shown to be superior as a pain reliever when compared to a regular bath of tap water.

> ### Core Question
> ||||||||||||||||||||||||||||||||||||||||
>
> *Can Yoga Help My Back Pain?*
>
> Yoga has long been considered an effective treatment for back pain. I've heard colleagues say that patients with back pain never practice yoga, and those who practice yoga never have back pain. My own review of the literature has been less convincing, however.
>
> One of the problems with discussing the benefits of yoga regarding back pain is that yoga comes in many forms; yoga is not one single thing, but many. That being said, there are elements of yoga, including flexibility, core strengthening, relaxation techniques, mood elevation, and self-efficacy, that undoubtedly contribute to improvement in back pain. Some of the Hidden Core Workout outlined in this book is derived from yoga, and incorporating more yoga certainly couldn't hurt.[10]

Willow Bark and Capsaicin Cream

The bark of the white willow tree (*Salix alba*) has pain-relieving properties similar to those of aspirin. It has an ingredient that's converted by the body into salicylic acid, known to lessen pain.

Capsaicin cream is derived from chili peppers. When applied topically, it creates heat and pain relief.

Both of these treatments are applied topically.

THE BIG S

Leaving the section of pain management leads us to the unavoidable, controversial, and often confusing discussion of surgery as treatment for back pain. If you've been exercising the hidden core, and have continued to make the Hidden Core Workout a part of your lifestyle while undergoing some of the pain management techniques and practices discussed in this chapter, you might still be wondering, "Am I a candidate for surgery?" And, "Where do I begin in this frightening and foreign process?"

I can't say that I haven't been looking forward to writing the next chapter, since first and foremost I'm a neuro*surgeon*. I have a plethora of information as well as opinions that I'm eager to share. This is my invitation to you to enter the private inner workings of the mind of a surgeon, if you dare to accept it.

The Gist

- When it comes to pain management, surgery isn't the *only* option and should rarely be the *first* option.

- There are many ways to manage pain, including medications, injections, pain procedures (using tools such as the dorsal column stimulator and the morphine pump), hands-on therapies, acupuncture, yoga, physical therapy, traction, and mattress selection.

SURGERY

A S A SURGEON who has just diagnosed a condition and recommended a treatment to a patient, I am asked many questions. Some are pointed and pragmatic; others, depending on the patient, are fueled by emotion and fear. There's one question, though—one I get a lot—that's motivated by the patient's desire to appeal to my human side (or at least to find out if I *have* one): "What would you tell your mother to do?"

It's a question I don't like to answer. Not only because I've never been able to tell my mother what to do, but because answering it influences the patient in a way I want to avoid. The question is often a signal to me that the patient is unable to decide. By asking this question, he or she may be looking for a shortcut. The problem with this is that it puts me, the "expert," rather than the patient, in the driver's seat.

My question for you, then, is, How much do you value your own instinct? I may be the expert on matters of the spine, but *you're* the expert on your own body. I'm not saying that my instinct won't help, but the ultimate decision needs to come from our *collaboration*.

Ideally, my recommendations will resonate with your instinct. If they don't, you need a different doctor. What's essential is that we communicate well enough to allow for this potential harmony to be fairly put to the test.

I'll begin this chapter on surgery with my personal views, experiences, and perceptions about surgery, based on the patients that I've treated (and not treated) over the last twenty years. I want to provide you with the rare opportunity to get "inside a surgeon's head." To go on a journey that will help you understand just how much the onus is on *you* (as scary as that may seem) when it comes to your health, while also assisting you in figuring out as much as you can about your surgeon's biases, instincts, and goals for your health.

I'll begin by unlocking the first secret, and it's a biggie: Just as you often leave a doctor's office with a strong impression—sometimes good and sometimes bad—I, too, often react to individual patients. The following is a description of "how I think" and "what I'm looking for" when I meet a patient.

First, I should tell you that I wake up every morning eager to go to work. This was true even during my exhausting residency. When I finished medical school, I had the sense that I'd already learned 90 percent of the entire subject matter of medicine. When I was a year into residency, this overconfidence had been replaced by the realization that I'd barely scratched the surface of the field of neurosurgery. I decided to completely immerse myself.

For the seven years after medical school I didn't pick up a newspaper or a novel; I avoided the "real world" completely. Now, when I look back, I don't recognize any of the music or movies that were produced or current events that took place during that time. I spent thousands upon thousands of hours assimilating a new body of information and learning the technical aspects of surgery, just as any apprentice does when learning a trade. (I know that there has been much discussion of overworked residents, but I can think of no other way to reach medical expertise outside of total dedication, however painful.) When I finished and resumed a social life, I distinctly remember feeling painfully awkward at cocktail parties because I had nothing to say; I'd had no life outside the hospital for an eternity.

The twenty years that followed were spent building a practice in neurosurgery. As is often the case, I realize in retrospect that what I thought several years ago I knew well, I now know much better! Such a realization is humbling and leads to a healthy skepticism of the methods I use and beliefs that I have today.

In my practice, I always balance two opposing forces: the desire to learn new ideas and techniques and the knowledge that putting them into practice subjects my patients to an inherent learning curve.

When I see a patient in my office, my strategy has always been simply to listen to what he or she has to say. As a diagnostician, I believe that the patient always "has the answer" and it's up to me to extract it. You may be surprised to hear that I make most diagnoses after only a few seconds of hearing the patient's history. The difficult part for me in these cases is teaching the patient what I believe the problem is, and why.

This teaching component ties into the necessary evolution of medicine discussed elsewhere in this book. Self-empowerment requires that my patients learn about and, ultimately, understand their condition. Once this is done, they must then take responsibility for their condition. My job is to be a diagnostician first and a teacher second. My final responsibility rests in removing myself so that my patients become autonomous.

HYPOTHETICALLY SPEAKING

Let's say you've made an appointment to see me. When you first come into my office, what I look for is a description of what you *feel*—what your body is telling you—not what you *think* is wrong. Oftentimes, when a patient believes deeply that something particular is wrong, it's hard to undo that belief as I explain my diagnosis and my recommendation regarding what (or what not) to do about it. In order to get the most bang for your buck, so to speak, when seeing a surgeon (or any diagnostician), try your best to present an unprejudiced depiction of what you've been experiencing. Editorializing is acceptable later, after I've had a chance to make a diagnosis.

Perhaps you've made your appointment to see me for a second opinion. Second opinions are an essential part of decision making for many patients. They're not a given, though. One thing to consider is whether having more than one point of view would be helpful to you, or would be potentially overwhelming. Some patients thrive on conflicting ideas and can use the contrast between them to their advantage, while others feel worse off with two different ideas and an associated inability to find a common ground. If you do see me for a second opinion, I prefer that you explicitly state that intention. I actually really enjoy offering a second opinion—I don't mind being *only* a consultant, as some patients fear—and find it a helpful way to ultimately teach and get across my own message. I look at it as a healthy challenge and as an introduction to a meaningful dialogue.

In the world of back pain, there are things that I automatically look for. Are you, the patient, embellishing your situation? Do you have a lawyer? Is there secondary gain? And yet I have to be very careful to not allow these extraneous contingencies to detract from what may be a significant and genuine problem. Again, honesty on your part, along with an uneditorialized version of events, goes a long way in allowing me to do my job in an unbiased way. If you have a problem, tell it like it is. The impact will not be lost.

A patient named Sara came to see me a few years ago. She'd had an injury at work and felt pain in one leg. When I examined her, I found weakness in all the muscles of that leg. This didn't match the MRI findings, and I wondered if she was embellishing the exam—in other words,

---

Core Concept
|||||||||||||||||||||||||||||||||||||||

While in the office with me, please don't tell me that you have a high tolerance for pain. Tolerance for pain does vary from patient to patient, although the threshold for pain nerves firing in response to a painful stimulus doesn't vary much. Any differences in tolerance are related to cultural differences and personal experiences. (Remember the brain's judicial function and the interpretive context of pain.)

The reason I ask you not to mention your "high tolerance" is that healthcare providers have a common reaction to that statement. It's our experience that when a patient makes such a declaration, almost invariably the exact opposite turns out to be true. So don't embarrass yourself; say nothing of your pain threshold.

---

exaggerating her weakness by giving less than 100 percent effort. I explained to her that I was concerned about offering her treatment without being able to account for this unexpected weakness. After she gained trust in me, she admitted to having embellished her weakness. Her motive was not to fake a problem, but to make sure that I took her problem seriously. She'd assumed that I would disregard her pain if there was nothing on the exam to confirm her complaints. She was surprised to learn that her efforts to substantiate her legitimate problem came close to undermining it instead.

I have to not only understand your pain, but also put it into the context of your typical routine. If you're seventy-five years old and have pain when you swing a golf club, I need to understand how important golf is to you. Every patient is unique; a limitation that's significant in one patient may be unimportant in another. For example, the seventy-five-year-old who wants to play golf may opt for an operation more readily than a less active patient.

Early on in taking a patient's history, I always try to sort out how much of the pain is in the back and how much is in the leg (or legs). This is an essential part of the history: Not only is the cause of leg pain easier to identify than that of back pain, but the treatment of leg pain is much more predictably successful, whether that treatment be physical therapy, pain management, or surgery.

I can't tell you how often patients come in to see me with a negative view of back surgery. It's important to recognize that this negativity is based on the results of surgery done to improve back pain as opposed to surgery aimed at leg pain. As you detail your history, be sure to specify how much of your pain is in the back and how much is in the leg. The relative level of each will play a significant role in my recommendations for you.

Furthermore, the more that the MRI or CT imaging can correlate with the specific nature of your leg pain, the better the potential results. In other words, if the MRI shows a piece of disc material pushing on the L5 nerve root, and you have leg pain (and only leg pain) that corresponds to the L5 nerve root territory, I can predict that results of treatment (whatever form you elect to pursue) will be good.

I'm keenly interested in whether your pain is related to your activities, and how it's related. In the golfer example above, I talked about needing to know about activities as a matter of context; here I'm trying to correlate specific activities to your pain. I like to think of pain as being either "mechanical," meaning predictably produced by a specific activity like swinging a tennis racquet, or "nonmechanical," meaning not predictably relieved by a specific *non*activity like lying down. In anticipating the potential success of surgery, there's a big difference between mechanical and nonmechanical pain. The former is much more treatable with surgery. Those who have pain all the time and in all positions fare worse with surgery than those who have pain with standing and complete relief with, for example, lying down.

Once I've concluded that your pain is mechanical, it's essential to understand the specific relation of your pain to when you're sitting, standing, and lying down. Lying down can be further broken down to lying supine (face up), lying prone, and lying on your side. You should also note whether bending your legs while supine helps the pain and whether turning from side to side hurts. These specific positions and movements help to identify the part of the spine that may be causing the pain. (Please refer to the section on the disc and the facet joints in chapter 5.)

When you come for a consultation, I'll want to evaluate your pain in conjunction with an MRI of the lumbar spine. There's a trend in this country to limit the "excessive" ordering of lumbar spine MRIs for back pain because of the test's "cost-ineffectiveness." And it's true that treating back pain *without* an imaging study is typically successful in acute cases, because of the favorable natural history of most acute back pain. In cases of more chronic back pain, however, I believe that MRIs are a helpful part of the diagnostic workup and should be integrated into the treatment plan, along with the history and the findings on the physical exam.

I often use the expression that "knowledge is power," and I believe that knowledge is particularly helpful in the treatment of back pain. For that reason, I want to be the *first* doctor who sees you. Again, there's a trend to utilize a generalist or a physician extender due to supposed cost-effectiveness, but in cases of back pain that have been persistent or intermittent over a long time, I believe that the most cost-effective encounter will be with a provider who can see the whole picture— which is to say, can not only take the history and do the exam, but read the MRI and select an appropriate treatment based on a working knowledge of *all* the various treatment options.

Once I've seen you and issued an opinion, I look for independence in you. I don't want to hear you say, "You're the doctor," or "Whatever you say." I like to be challenged. One thing that separates me from some of the other healthcare providers is that my goal for you is independence. As opposed to therapists, chiropractors, pain management doctors, and certain other healthcare providers, I and my fellow surgeons do best by seeing you once or twice and setting you on the right path.

With most other treatments, in contrast, the more dependent you are, the better the provider—the physical therapist, say, or the chiropractor—does from a financial point of view. The same can be said with the treatment of pain with medications. The longer you stay on the medications, the happier the pharmaceutical industry is.

When I refer you to physical therapy or to a chiropractor, therefore, I expect you to learn about yourself and the treatment so that you can ultimately self-administer, rather than seeking to be passively healed. Therapy is a medium by which *you* heal *yourself.* So when you say to me, "You're the doctor," or "Whatever you say, Doc," I worry that you'll never take an active role in your healing. Even after I operate (if that's our decision), if you need follow-on physical therapy or exercise, your passive attitude will only impede the healing and strengthening process.

If I order a test, it's up to *you* to ask about the results and not up to me to remember to give them to you. It's essential that you take this active role in compiling the necessary information for diagnosis and in monitoring the success of your treatment. I want you to succeed almost as much as you want to succeed, but I can only be a helpful teacher or resource. I can't be your motivator or your driving force. When you're with me, you have my full attention, but when you leave, the next patient has my full attention. Taking an active role maximizes your chances of success.

Roth's R$_X$: Don't put your body in anyone's hands without being an active participant in the process. Facilitate a positive relationship between you and your healthcare provider by being interested in achieving autonomy. This will ultimately expedite the strengthening process after surgery.

Please don't let your family and friends participate too much in your assessments. They'll influence you unduly with anecdotes that involve patients who have underlying pathologies that are far different from yours. Unless your advisers have actually perused your MRI and the MRI of the other patient(s) on which they're basing their advice, they shouldn't be suggesting a comparison treatment. The ultimate analysis is yours and only yours. If you need help in judging the relative nature of your improvement, I suggest that you use me to provide that prospective, because I'll compare apples to apples, which your friends and family will be unable to do.

Finally, always view your problem through an expanded horizon. Back pain is a part of life. This is to say, not only is it a ubiquitous problem, but it's a dynamic problem that never really comes to an end. Even the straightforward herniated disc that's effectively treated with surgery to remove the herniated disc fragment doesn't represent the end of the story. There's always a life lesson to be learned. Why did the disc herniation occur in the first place? What can you do to prevent another disc herniation? Are there genetic issues? Are there modifications that need to be made in your activities, in your diet, in your expectations? Your success will be defined not only in the present, but in your ability to adapt over time. I look for this sense of patience and equanimity in you.

Hidden Truth 19: Surgery Is Merely a Preparation
for Physical Therapy!

A patient in his seventies complained of bilateral leg pain and back pain during his first office visit. He told me that he was able to walk for only one to two minutes before having to stop. Because he could control the pain by sitting down, he wasn't interested in surgery. He had been treated with epidural steroid injections and physical therapy in the past, with only a small amount of benefit. He felt stronger and more flexible with the therapy, but he had the same pain with walking. The injections gave him only temporary relief from back and leg pain; furthermore, as is usually the case with narcotics, the treatment became less effective with each injection.

Because the pain had been so persistent, he came to my office to discuss surgery. His primary-care doctor, his friends, and his family had all told him to avoid surgery because of his advanced age. In addition, he had heard of many people who had gone through back surgery for similar complaints, only to end up with more pain.

This case illustrates a classic situation that our aging population frequently goes through. The patient was so focused on the pain that he wasn't fully aware of what he'd lost in terms of his daily repertoire of activity. He'd convinced himself that he didn't *like* shopping or traveling. What he didn't fully realize was that it was the *walking* that he was avoiding, and not the shopping or traveling. Only by looking back at a typical day over the past several years and comparing it with his current daily routine was he able to see how much his activity had been curtailed. This is typical of spinal stenosis, as I noted earlier. The effects are insidious and thus less noticeable. By the time the different lifestyle is evident, the curtailment has permeated the patient's sense of what he or she enjoys in a way that's hard to restore. In addition, the patient's general stamina and conditioning suffer months or years of slow and steady decline.

Even if a stenosis patient considers a surgical reprieve, his family, friends, or healthcare provider may discourage it. This discouragement would be based on what? Old age? Patients are often surprised to find out that the average age of surgery for spinal stenosis is well into the seventies. They also may be surprised that the general impressions of how poor the results of spine surgery are don't necessarily apply to this group of patients. In fact, the majority of stenosis patients end up enabled, with more ability to walk and do activities of daily living. Better yet, in most cases these positive changes are apparent in less than two weeks.

Again, the message here is that spinal stenosis surgery works, in general, because it's not so much designed to remove pain as it is to enable the patient and promote health through exercise.

Roth's R_X: Surgery works best when it enables activity. This allows for the patient to exercise and mitigate the pain.

SO, YOU'RE THINKING ABOUT SURGERY . . .

Among surgeons who operate on the brain, it's said that "the wheat is separated from the chaff" in terms of their technical prowess. Among spine surgeons, that separation is made on the basis of decision-making prowess. Isn't that ironic? Spine surgery is a more intellectual pursuit than brain surgery! Perhaps the familiar cliché should be changed to "It doesn't take a spine surgeon to . . ."

If you reach the point where you're contemplating surgery, it's imperative that your discussions with the surgeon include not only a technical explanation for the procedure that the surgeon is recommending, but also an explanation of the decision process and rationale for the recommended surgery, which is far more difficult to communicate. Regrettably, most surgeons want to tell you what they're going to do to you, but not explain why they want to do it.

This section of the book is designed not to help you find the "right" procedure to have, but rather to help you gain a general education on the philosophy of surgery, which will help you communicate with your surgeon. As Albert Einstein said about education, it's what's left over when all that was learned in school has been forgotten. Your "education" here will not be the knowledge of the individual procedures, but the rationale that indicates them.

I'm well aware of the general negative perception of surgery in the community. The vast majority of patients I see are biased in a negative way at the outset. It's very common for a patient to say to me that he or she knows someone who had surgery and is now "in agony all the time" or is "tied to a wheelchair." When I try to pursue details regarding these (in my patients' words) destroyed or miserable patients, it becomes clear that most of the information is secondhand—those helpful friends and relatives again!—and probably exaggerated. That being said, there's a lot of bad surgery performed in this country, and there are a lot of bad outcomes, justifiably leading to the bad reputation that surgery holds.

But there are also plenty of success stories, particularly when the right patient gets the appropriate procedure—and when that procedure is executed in the correct way. Again, it all comes down to starting your process with a specialist. This is why I believe that the proper starting point for any back pain sufferer is with a surgeon.

This is obviously a biased opinion, of course. There are certainly other providers who possess the ability to discuss all aspects of the case. However, the training and experience of surgeons puts us uniquely into this position. It's up to us to overcome the natural bias of looking at patients *first* as potential surgical candidates and instead to apply our knowledge to outlining the most cost-effective and efficient solution to your pain and your unique presentation.

Core Concept

Medicine is an art more than a science. Accordingly, the decision for surgery often requires a comparison of different shades of gray. There are nuances, and one should expect the decision to be difficult. If it seems really simple, consider the possibility that you're being fed a watered-down explanation. In addition, if it seems "too good to be true," it probably is. *All* surgical decisions for back pain must be individualized. Even if two patients have the same MRI findings and the same symptoms, the treatment may be different. Surgery decisions need to consider not only the pathology on the MRI, but the body type and condition, the age, the activity routine, and the expectations that you, the patient, present. Surgery is not a one-size-fits-all solution.

HOW TO CHOOSE A BACK SURGEON

Would you be surprised to learn that I have trouble discerning the level of talent among my surgical colleagues? Some surgeons are good at certain procedures and yet not as good at others. Some surgeons are great one day and not as great the next day. What makes a surgeon great anyway? Is it the hand dexterity? Is it the speed at which the case moves? And how about the ultimate results—how do you judge those? Do you focus on patient satisfaction, or are there more objective criteria?

The bottom line is that there are no universal criteria by which to rate surgeons. Individual surgeons certainly have a reputation, but what is that really based on? Is it their personality? Their popularity with referring professionals? You, as the patient, have little ability to find out what you'd really like to know. It's not as if a surgeon can (or would) invite you into the operating room for a sneak preview.

How do you decide, then, on your surgeon? To some extent, you'll need to trust your instinct. It's perfectly fine to do due diligence and thoroughly research your surgeon in any way you can, but at some point you must relinquish the idea that you'll ever arrive at an unequivocal truth. Even if you could visit the operating room and watch several surgeons at work, it would be difficult—especially for you, as a layperson—to know which one would be the correct choice for you. I say this not to create despair, but rather to provide encouragement in the power your instinct can hold.

Beyond what your instinct tells you about a surgeon, you also need to decide between a neurosurgeon and an orthopedic spine surgeon. Although the approaches and sensibilities of the training differ slightly between the two specialties, it's primarily the individual personality and personal experience, not the title, that defines and distinguishes each surgeon.

If you were to ask me, I would naturally give a biased comparison of the training of each. In general, I believe that most neurosurgeons have a more extensive training in the spine than orthopedic spine surgeons.

In fact, organized neurosurgery, in the form of the American Association of Neurological Surgeons, doesn't acknowledge spine fellowship
training, feeling that it is not a necessary addition to achieve compe-
tence.

The distinction between surgical types isn't as crucial as one might
expect, however. Any surgeon who has been in practice for some time
has transcended the particular background and training, for the most
part. Again, remember that medicine in general, and spine surgery
specifically, is more an art than a science. Judge your surgeon as an
artist and as a person, as much as a technician. I often hear patients
say, "I don't care what kind of personality my surgeon has; I just want
him to be technically sound." I strongly take issue with this argument,
because there's much more to surgery than the technical exercise that
occurs in the operating room.

Few patients have the energy, ability, or confidence to incorporate
all of the nuances required to make a truly informed decision about
back treatment. They rely, rather, on their instinct, which I endorse, as
noted earlier. In addition, it turns out that individuals are often pre-
disposed to a particular type of decision. Some of us are comfortable
with intervention, for example, while others believe in the body's innate
capacity to heal. Some of us are comfortable following a surgeon's
advice, while others use the experience of a friend or family member
as the primary basis for their decision. Few of us engage in the pains-
taking process that's necessary to make the best decision.[1]

HOW TO DECIDE WHICH SURGERY (IF ANY) TO HAVE

More important than which surgeon you choose is the choice of whether
or not to have surgery, and which particular surgery to opt for. I'll mention some generalities that might be helpful for you to consider as you
make your choice.

Are you contemplating surgery primarily for back pain or for leg pain? This is the point that decisions about lumbar spine surgery must start with. In general, the results for the treatment of leg pain are much better than those for back pain, as we've seen. The surgeon may tell you that there's, say, a 90 percent chance of pain relief with a certain type of surgery, but he or she may be referring only to leg pain, not to back pain. If you have both, it's important to find out what the percentage for improvement is for back pain and for leg pain, separately.

It's important to know not only what the success rate is, but also how your surgeon defines success. You must realize, of course, that the percentages your surgeon gives you are only a rough, educated guess. There's a body of literature that helps make the guess somewhat of an educated guess, but it's a guess nonetheless.

Furthermore, surgeons are prone to a couple *external* biases that make interpreting prospective results difficult: Some patients don't want to disappoint the surgeon (or are shy about sharing their own disappointment) and thus don't report accurately on how they're feeling, while other patients are overly optimistic initially and fail to give the surgeon true feedback over time—*both* distortions potentially leading to a falsely optimistic outlook. Another external bias can result in the surgeon's being overly pessimistic: One of the frustrations of being a surgeon is that your successes leave your practice quickly because they no longer need you, while your failures continue to come back for help. This tends to increase the percentage of failures relative to successes that the surgeon sees each day.

I define success not in terms of pain resolution, for I think that pain resolution is often an unrealistic goal. Rather, I define success as a patient answering the question, "Are you glad you had the surgery?" with a definitive "Yes." I do my best to use objective statistics as a guide in providing percentages, but I know that these are incomplete at best.

The next consideration when deciding on surgery is how the limitations imposed after surgery will affect your specific plans for work,

Core Concept
||||||||||||||||||||||||||||||||||||||

Always ask your surgeon to explain the natural history of your problem—that is, the projected course of the problem if it isn't treated. Patients routinely ask me, "What do I have?" or "What's the treatment?" They ask me about potential outcomes and complications, but seldom do they ask, "What happens if I do nothing?" This is an essential piece of information as you make your decision.

It has always been my preference to see the patient prior to any treatment so that I can provide the patient with an overview of the natural history of his or her condition, review potential treatments, and select the best starting point and pathway. It's rare for healthcare providers other than surgeons to be able to read the MRI, examine the patient, and discuss *all* possible options.

family life, and activities of daily living. You should ask when you'll be able to drive again, when you'll be able to return to work, when you'll be able to walk, and when you'll be able to exercise. It's helpful to keep a brief diary of your daily activities *before* consulting with the surgeon so that a return to the important activities can be specifically addressed during your presurgical visit.

When discussing complications, it's important that the patient learn what can happen in theory, but the *focus* should be on the more common issues. I often tell patients that contemplating surgery is analogous to preparing for a plane flight. It's more meaningful to focus on the cost of the tickets, or on whether it will be a nonstop flight, than on whether the plane might crash. For back surgery, the main complication that you'll face will be failure to improve, not the many more rare complications that are theoretically possible.

Your decision should thus focus first and foremost on the chance of improvement; you should weigh this against the probability of lack of improvement or worsening, rather than against the potential rare injury to nerve roots, spinal fluid leak, infection, and so on. Focusing on the rare complications can be done after you've established some direction and momentum in the decision-making process. If you focus initially on the unlikely possibility of, for example, paralysis, that will detract from the more relevant concerns.

THE SECOND OPINION

In general, getting a second opinion is a good idea. However, as I mentioned above, a second opinion isn't for everyone. There are two main reasons to get a second opinion: to decide on which surgery to do, and to shop around for another surgeon. You should have in mind *why* you're seeking a second opinion. Some patients are capable of integrating the opinions of more than one surgeon and benefiting from the experience, while other patients are immobilized by the decision-making process. As the process becomes more complex, with added opinions, that latter patient's state of mind gets worse. Are you comfortable contrasting differing options and approaches prior to getting a second opinion? Will more information be helpful or overwhelming? Finally, some people seek out second or third opinions until the opinion matches what they've already decided they want. This is a really bad reason to look for another opinion.

A second opinion is valid only if it's offered and received with an open mind. If there's something about the surgeon offering the second opinion that turns you off so that you're unable to "hear" what that surgeon is saying, the second opinion is useless. Your instinct is telling you that you should either find another second opinion or abandon the idea of a second opinion.

As I stated earlier, even though it's essential that you attempt to understand any proposed surgery (and the nuances of the surgeon's decision-making process), it's also important to understand that, ultimately, you'll have to trust the surgeon. If that trust isn't there, a second opinion is not only helpful, it's a necessity. Your gut will be your guide.

HOW WILL YOU PROGRESS AFTER THE OPERATION?

Just as surgeons shouldn't be judged on their technique alone, but also on their selection process and indications for surgery, their management of patients in the postoperative period is worthy of serious scrutiny. As is the case with so many facets of medicine, there's no definitive answer for how to progress the postoperative patient back to activities of daily life; surgeons vary greatly in their approach.

Conceptually, the decision-making process regarding the resumption of various activities weighs the relative risk of a possible setback against the obvious benefits of a return to normalcy. In the case of the microdiscectomy, this tension is particularly poignant. This procedure has a documented reoccurrence rate of 5 to 10 percent, which is relatively high. The strength of the healing tissues, moreover, doesn't reach a high percentage of its ultimate strength until around six weeks. For these reasons, many surgeons opt to advise patients to "take it easy," encouraging them to limit lifting, sitting, and repetitive bending to allow damaged tissue to become more robust and near its final strength.

Contrast this to the habits of many surgeons in Europe, who tend to mobilize their patients more quickly. Their decision is based on a fear of scar tissue on the nerve roots, a condition called epidural fibrosis, which some consider an occasional cause of postoperative pain.

It's important to get your surgeon's view and philosophy on this subject and to see if it resonates with you. You could probably guess that I tend to mobilize my patients quickly. I individualize this judg-

> ## Core Question
> ||||||||||||||||||||||||||||||||||||||||||
>
> *Will I Be "Scarred" by Scar Tissue?*
>
> Scar tissue is one of the most controversial concepts in the world of spine surgery. Any time human tissue is cut—whether superficial tissue (the skin) or internal tissue (e.g., the heart)—scar tissue will form. In spine surgery, however, the issue of scar tissue formation has taken on a life of its own. Scar tissue is commonly invoked as a source of pain after surgery. Prior to surgery, I'm frequently asked about scar tissue by concerned patients.
>
> Although I have no doubt that there are occasions in which scarring of the nerve root after surgery plays a part in postoperative pain, most of the time scar tissue is unfairly ascribed as a cause. More likely, the pain is related to an aspect of the surgical technique—for example, an incompletely decompressed nerve. Scar tissue is a convenient scapegoat that has been propagated by surgeons as a way to blame the patient and his or her healing pattern, rather than the way the surgery was executed.

ment based on the patient and the intraoperative findings, though. My rationale isn't so much a fear of epidural fibrosis, but the belief that scar tissue is a live entity that can be "molded" and strengthened by properly stressing it. Rather than just letting the scar tissue strengthen, I act on my belief that it can be made better by properly stressing it *while* it strengthens.

THE BIG THREE

There are a host of different surgical procedures for various back and leg ailments. While I realize that you can easily go on the Internet to

learn more about them, I'll highlight what I refer to as the Big Three—
the most common surgical treatments that I conduct (and the ones that
cause the most anxiety and confusion among my patients). Once you
know about these, you can begin to apply the philosophies discussed
above to your decision-making process.

Hidden Truth 20: Minimally Invasive Can Be Maximally Evasive!

When used in medicine, the label "invasive" refers to how much your
body is disrupted or compromised. "Minimally invasive," when used
to describe surgery, suggests that your body will have little in the way
of disruption or compromise. "Minimally invasive surgery" is a term
that has gained popularity of late, to such an extent that surgeons have
started to use it as a marketing tool. After all, who wouldn't opt for the
least possible damage? The pairing of "new" and "minimally invasive"
is especially persuasive: Surgeons like to pitch a "newer" procedure
(available instead of a "traditional" procedure) that is also "less
invasive"—less of an ordeal for the patient to go through—but, at the
same time, can be expected to yield a similar efficacy.

In surgery of the spine, we prefer the term "minimal access" rather
than "minimally invasive" because it more accurately represents a
procedure that's gentler, but equally efficacious. We substitute the word
"access" for "invasive" because many of the procedures we do *are* invasive. These procedures disrupt and compromise the patient, yes; but
they're performed with minimal effects on those tissues that need to
be compromised in performing the operation. When contemplating a
minimally invasive or minimal access procedure, the patient must
determine whether the newer treatment is equally *effective*. A gentler
procedure that accomplishes less isn't necessarily the best option.

As noted, many of the surgical procedures done on the spine are
invasive. A fusion, for example, is an invasive procedure—no matter
how it's done. Surfaces of bone are made to bleed, and donor bone is

placed between those bleeding surfaces with the hope of joining two structures that are supposed to be separate and mobile. How the structures are accessed in terms of incisional length, muscle retraction, and disruption and time of surgery all determine whether the access has been minimalized. Minimal access can lead to quicker recovery and less postoperative pain.

Innovations in spine surgery technology have increased the number of surgeries that qualify as minimal access. Introduction of the operating microscope and the high-speed precision drill, for instance, have revolutionized spine surgery. The microscope provides unparalleled magnification and lighting along with anatomical detail that has fundamentally changed what surgeons are able to see. The new drills allow for bone to be removed precisely to maximize visualization and minimize weakening of the bones or joints.

Roth's R$_X$: Minimally invasive surgery is great as
long as there's no compromise in the efficacy.

Microdiscectomy

Typically performed to alleviate a herniated lumbar disc, a microdiscectomy is actually more effective for treating leg pain than treating lower back pain. Surgeons recommend it for both ailments, however. Microdiscectomy is the removal of a piece of disc that's irritating a nerve root. The prefix "micro" suggests that the procedure is done under magnification and through a small incision. There is variability among surgeons as to the size of the incision made and the type of magnification utilized. In my opinion, the optimal tool for doing this procedure is the operating microscope. This microscope provides more magnification, better optics, and better lighting than the alternatives (the loupe and the endoscope). Surprisingly, my guess is that the majority of discectomies are done without the microscope.

There are many additional variables in the execution of the micro-discectomy. Some surgeons split the muscles rather than retract en route to the laminae (the bone forming the dorsal wall of the spinal canal), for example. Some surgeons routinely remove more bone than others. Some remove more of the facet joint than others to gain access. The amount of disc material removed also varies: Some surgeons remove only the offending fragment of disc, while others do an aggressive removal of disc material that has not herniated. The literature doesn't provide any proof that there's a superior method of doing a discectomy. It's reasonable, though, to suggest that minimizing the damage done to the muscles and joints in exposing the herniated disc likely leads to less pain and a quicker recovery. This supposition is at the heart of minimal access surgery.

Just as there's variability in the actual procedure, there's variability in the *indications* for microdiscectomy. Some surgeons see the predominance of leg pain over back pain to be necessary to recommend the procedure, while others operate on patients even with the predominance of back pain.

Similarly, there's variability in judging what is sufficient conservative care—that is, nonsurgical care done before surgery is recommended. Some surgeons prescribe and supervise the type of therapy done and the nature of any injection treatment administered. Some ask specific questions about not only the duration and intensity of the pain, but how the pain affects the patient on a day-to-day basis. Others are less discerning. I'm one to scrutinize the therapy and the exact nature of the pain management prior to suggesting surgery. It's not prudent to indicate surgery because a patient has "failed" conservative treatment if the nature of that conservative treatment isn't fully understood.

Questions to ask your surgeon regarding any proposed discectomy:
1. How many microdiscectomies have you done?
2. Do you use a microscope?
3. How much bone and facet joint do you remove?

4. How much disc do you remove?

5. How do you protect the muscles?

Of course, to many of these questions you won't know what the right answer is. I've got news for you. Neither do I! Nor does your surgeon! By asking these questions, though, you'll gain insight into the philosophical approach of your surgeon and strengthen your convictions regarding your ultimate decision. You should look for a surgeon who has done at least hundreds of the procedure. I think the microscope is a must; precision is lost with the alternative tools. The other questions will force a dialogue, which will be helpful.

Fusion

As I mentioned earlier, my world is replete with stories that begin, "I know someone who had a fusion and now is a disaster." It may surprise you to hear that the terrible reputation of fusion surgery is well earned! That being said, there's an appropriate time and place for fusion surgery.

Fusion is designed to stop the motion between two mobile segments of the spine by creating a bridge of bone. This bridge of bone, which solidifies over time from the implantation of the donor bone, is live tissue with its own blood supply. Like any bone, it can strengthen and be modified in its shape over time. The perception of fusion for most people involves the placement of metallic hardware into the bones; and although this is often the case, this hardware is there only to facilitate the bony fusion (holding the implanted bone in place until the bones have knit together). The hardware doesn't suffice to permanently eliminate motion between two spinal segments unless there's a biological bridge that forms. No matter how strong the metal implant is, it eventually loosens if there's no bony fusion.

Most fusions are done to eliminate pain. Conceptually, the surgeon uses the history, physical exam, and imaging studies to implicate a particular segment of the spine as a pain generator and then fuses this segment. This seems simple, but it's more difficult than it sounds.

Fusions fail for two main reasons: Either the implicated segment wasn't the pain generator (or not the *sole* pain generator), or the surgery didn't adequately fuse the implicated segment. It's the former, the inability to adequately localize the source of pain, that most commonly results in failure. Even in cases where there's only one significant abnormality seen in the spine on imaging studies, in many cases that lone abnormality isn't solely responsible for the pain. This finding arises from the complex nature of pain, which I've addressed throughout the book. As a patient contemplating a fusion operation, you must understand how the surgeon has selected which segment or segments to fuse, as well as how the surgeon will accomplish the fusion.

Localizing the segment of pain generation is a complex process. The surgeon typically integrates the CT scan, X-ray, or MRI findings with the clinical nature of the pain; he or she may also incorporate procedures designed to provoke the pain, or to temporarily relieve the pain, through nerve or facet injection. In general, the more tests and findings that implicate the same specific segment of the spine, the higher the likelihood of success.

Accomplishing the fusion can be achieved via a variety of approaches. The current literature provides surgeons little guidance in understanding which procedure is best in each particular case. Although I'm an advocate for educating you as completely as possible, this complicated aspect of decision making is even farther toward art on the art-science continuum than the other material we've been considering. The scientific literature on fusion is, simply, incomplete. Obviously, you should make an effort to understand the nuances of the ultimate decision, but of all the conceptual areas that you'll try to embrace in the contemplation of surgery, this is the one area where you'll have to relinquish control and simply trust the surgeon.

Salvatore is a fifty-one-year-old man who came to me after many years of episodes of low back pain. He also experienced occasional right leg pain. He'd had a disc herniation operation in his thirties with good results, but he felt that he'd never been "quite right" since. He'd also tried several programs of physical therapy, but he'd had unsustainable improvements. He felt that he was taking too much ibuprofen for his pain. In retrospect, after being questioned in my office, he admitted to having given up some of the activities that he loved— specifically, golf and running. He noted that these activities invariably brought on pain that typically lasted for a few days and were thus "not worth it."

When I examined him, he had intact strength and sensation. His flexibility was diminished by tight hamstrings, and his range of motion with flexion was diminished in the back. The MRI of his lumbar spine revealed an isolated problem at the L5–S1 disc space (the bottom disc of the spine). There was no nerve root compression, but the disc had lost height and water content. X-rays done of the lumbar spine in flexion and extension showed several millimeters of motion between flexion and extension. I explained to him that the findings on the MRI and on the X-rays suggested, but didn't prove, that the L5–S1 disc space abnormality was the generator of his pain.

When he heard the word "fusion" as my suggested treatment, he was quick to state that he would rather "live with the pain" than be operated on, because (he told me) everyone he knew who'd gone through a fusion had either not improved or had felt even worse.

Taking all this into account, I gave Salvatore the option of a minimal access fusion at L5–S1. This approach had the advantage of nearly no muscle disruption. After considerable discussion and thought, he opted for that approach. Once healed, he was able to return to running and golf and had far fewer of his low back pain exacerbations.

I'm aware that fusion is generally regarded as a four-letter word. This reflects more the misuse of the fusion operation than the fusion operation itself. The most common fusions performed in the United States are done for degenerative disc disease, which happens to be the one fusion operation *without* good evidence-based medicine to support its utility. This is an operation whose predicted success rate is often in the 50 percent range. That means that one-half of the patients who undergo this operation fail to gain significant benefit!

Obviously, an operation with a 50 percent success rate leaves a large number of people unsatisfied. When this is coupled with the frequency that the operation is performed, it leaves a lot of unsatisfied patients walking around complaining about their "failed" surgery. I always tell patients that I'm hesitant to do the operation, because no matter how strongly I reinforce the possibility of failure prior to the operation, our preoperative conversation will be forgotten. The patient will then complain to friends and family about persistent pain, all with my name associated with their experience.

There is, however, a subset of patients like Salvatore who find relief in the procedure. If surgeons would refrain from operating on the marginally indicated cases, that would go a long way toward improving the reputation of the procedure.

Roth's R$_X$: Though performed too much and often for the wrong reasons, fusion does provide successes to balance the downside. If you're considering a fusion, factor in the surgeon's rationale for doing the procedure.

Decompression

Like the microdiscectomy, decompression involves the removal of either hypertrophic or misplaced spinal tissue that's compressing a nerve or nerves. The two procedures differ in that while the microdiscectomy is primarily the removal of disc material, the decompression is primarily the removal of hypertrophic bone and ligament.

The label *decompression* is used interchangeably with such terms as *laminectomy, laminotomy, unroofing, cleaning out,* and many others. The fact that the terminology isn't consistently applied makes the matter more confusing for patients.

The same questions are pertinent to the decompression as to the microdiscectomy. I would recommend that you ask your surgeon the following: How much tissue is to be removed? Will a microscope be used? How are the facet joints protected? How many have you done? And so on.

One topic that should be added for the discussion of decompression is whether the "midline"—the spinous processes and their connecting ligaments—will be "preserved." Preservation of the midline is a nuance of decompression that involves the use of a less invasive, but technically more challenging, methodology. This issue is important, because preserving the spinous processes helps ensure the structural integrity of the spine. (Put another way, removal of the spinous processes deprives the spine of some of its support.)

Decompression isn't a good alternative for all patients, but it is advantageous for some. If you're contemplating this surgery and have a reasonable understanding of what your surgeon is proposing, the question of midline preservation would be a subtle technical matter to discuss. Like many of the questions I've suggested, there's no one correct answer. The question will create dialogue, which will help you elicit information and develop an opinion.

Surgery may be avoidable if you've been using the Hidden Core Workout. At times, though—for some people, in some circumstances—it's *un*avoidable. If you're one of those cases, don't think of surgery as a "solution." Using the philosophy that I hope to have instilled in you, you must think of surgery as a necessary step to allow you to begin the healing process.

The Gist

- Sometimes surgery is necessary, and may even be the first choice of treatment.

- Focusing more on the philosophy of a surgeon rather than on the technical parts of the surgery will help you elicit vital information about your treatment and healing process.

- In the spirit of self-sufficiency, think of surgery as merely a preparation for physical therapy.

CHAPTER 8

THE BACK GENOME

THIS BOOK has considered back pain from the philosophical perspective that most current conceptions of back pain are not only wrong, but detrimental. Friedrich Nietzsche once said, "Convictions are more dangerous foes of the truth than lies." Our beliefs that we need to find something "broken" and fix it, to rest when we're in pain, and to rely on outsiders to advise us about what's best are the type of convictions that I contend are hurting your back more than plain lies would.

Incorporating philosophical considerations like the one above, *The End of Back Pain* offers a perspective that's practical, empowering, and actionable in its approach to conceptualizing pain and mitigating it. It's my hope that you, as a reader, have lost some of your dangerous convictions and now have a greater understanding of your back pain and your options for improved back health.

I hope that you now understand how a diagnosis, and sometimes even the language used to justify that diagnosis, can take on a life of its own and actually affect the amount of pain you feel.

I hope that you *interpret* pain differently. For example, I hope that you understand that the state of mind you're in at the time the pain starts or increases is as important as the so-called "generator" of the pain. I hope you also understand that back pain arises in the brain, even in the straightforward case of a large disc herniation. This knowledge doesn't serve to trivialize pain, but rather to put pain in a different *context*—one that offers a new optimism along with additional potential methods of intervention.

I hope that you didn't survey the exercises of the Hidden Core Workout without also trying to learn the underlying anatomy and the rationalization of what the exercises are trying to accomplish.

Finally, I hope that your long-term expectations are to diminish the frequency, intensity, and duration of the inevitable occurrences of back pain, and *not* to eliminate back pain.

MOVING AHEAD

Much of this book was designed to discourage you from looking for a quick fix. One of the many parts of my job as a surgeon that I hadn't anticipated was the role of "life coach." I often spend as much time trying to instill a sense of realistic expectation into my patients as I spend on educating them on the anatomy and physiology of their back.

Patients often come into the office expecting a solution to their pain. Before we compare different treatment options, I always seek to clarify what a solution to pain actually is, in reality. And many times, they don't like it. "Time," I say, or "Nothing." Worse yet, "Pain is normal." I say these things to people looking at me with emptiness in their eyes, as if I'd just told them there was no Santa Claus. It pains me, as a doctor who took the Hippocratic Oath to "first do no harm," to see people seem so helpless and resentful when I share these realities with them.

My personal experience with patients who can't accept that they don't have to do anything for their back except work it, strengthen their hidden core, and gain a new healthy perspective on pain has compelled me to search for more tangible ways that the healthcare system can facilitate these large goals. After all, as discussed at the outset, we have many long-standing, pervasive cultural influences to take down, and we won't do it unless there's an empirically effective way to save us from the same expensive, less-than-satisfactory results offered today through the business of back pain. Albert Einstein described insanity as doing the same thing over and over again and expecting different results. That label could be applied to healthcare as it pertains to back pain.

So, where are you now, and where are you heading? Are you stuck in a sort of back pain quicksand, desperate for someone to hand you a branch to help pull you out? If so, good, because I have some unique ideas for you.

In Greek mythology, one of Apollo's sons was named Asclepius, and he was responsible for the health of mortals. He had two daughters named Hygeia and Panacea who, respectively, promoted health by washing patients (hygiene) and treating disease once it occurred (panacea, or cure-all). Clearly, our current medical system has largely followed the path of Panacea. Progress in this regard has been spectacular, but also spectacularly expensive. The idea of treating disease has led us to some powerful weapons, including antibiotics, chemotherapeutic agents, and cutting-edge surgical technologies. These innovations have brought not only the opportunity to cure some diseases, but an enormous price tag—once that's increasing at an unsustainable rate. Emphasis on promotion of health, on the other hand (rather than treatment of disease), has been shown to be cost-effective across many settings.

In the treatment of back pain, understanding the distinction between promotion of health and treatment of disease is paramount. It's the reason that I propose exercise as the primary treatment of back pain. It's also why I joke (only partly in jest) that surgery is merely a preparation for physical therapy. The point is that even surgery can be thought of as a facilitator of health promotion.

As medicine goes through its necessary restructuring process, one that has been made imperative by the need to control costs, I'm certain that the treatment of back pain will be part of that transition.

One of the fundamental changes will involve a shift of decision-making responsibility from the healthcare providers to the patients. This shift will not be mandated, but will occur naturally as the current trend of Internet-based research continues to increase. This shift of patient-driven care will be accompanied by a transition from the current system of disease treatment to a system of health promotion. Although there may be some mandates for this transition, it too will largely occur simply due to its demonstrated cost-effectiveness. These two transitions will be made possible by the creation of an online repository for what I call the "back genome."

THE BACK GENOME

In its original genetics context, a genome is the entirety of an organism's hereditary information; each person has a unique genome. You may have heard of the human genome project, which has been carried out over the past twenty years in an effort to map out the entire genetic code that's written in human DNA. This knowledge will undoubtedly serve to provide ideas, preventions, and treatments for a variety of disease processes.

The back genome is a related concept, insofar as it seeks to identify each person as an individual and unique (or "niche") back pain sufferer. This precision doesn't exist today, but it's a realistic possibility due to the technology now available, such as the Internet, smart phones, and system-based software that can manipulate enormous amounts of data.

Today's model, in contrast, is antiquated and obsolescent. It involves an almost arbitrary starting point for each patient. From there, an expert creates a diagnosis and treatment plan, both of which are inevitably influenced by that expert's subjective interpretation of the literature, limited experience, and inherent bias rooted in mercenary needs. With the help of the Internet, expertise in medicine will become a collaborative process. Diagnosis will come not from a single expert, but from simultaneous input of a database (which will define a "niche" presentation of back pain) and the interpretation and direction of an appropriate expert. Both healthcare providers and patients alike will learn to function in this medium. The Canadian philosopher Marshall McLuhan stated that "the medium is the message" in his 1962 book *The Gutenberg Galaxy.* What he suggested by that linkage is that as media evolves, so do our cognitive processes—much in the way our cognitive processes are tied into our physical bodies (that embodied cognition we talked about earlier). The Internet has made possible a new method of diagnosis and treatment. It's up to us to adapt to it.

Before discussing how this data could be acquired or how it pertains to a genome, let's explore what I mean by "niche" back pain presentation. In his book *The Long Tail,* provocative author Chris Anderson describes the emergence of "niche" cultural tastes that the Internet has facilitated.[1] In music, for example, many of us are accustomed to passively listening to radio stations and passively coming to enjoy a percentage of the songs we hear. We may, in turn, buy the songs that we like and thus slowly build a collection at home. The Internet has already played a part in this endeavor: The majority of music is bought over the Internet now.

In addition to this "passive" form of music acquisition, we may be more "active" and choose to visit certain stations based on the music selection provided. The Internet takes choice to a different level, however, allowing us to seek out music that's *likely* to be something that we would enjoy. This "active" pursuit—with the effort done by computer technology—lies in searching for similarities in the structure of the music that we like. It's no accident that the Internet radio station called Pandora, which introduces new music to each individual user based on that music's structural similarity to other selections enjoyed by the individual, refers to itself as the "music genome project."

In the past, the choice of what would be played on the radio was made by the DJs employed by any given radio station. Even before that choice-point, though, artists had to get over a hurdle: They couldn't even be considered by the DJs without a recording company deciding that they were worthwhile. In both of these cases, it wasn't you, the listener, who decided what was going to be played, but some "expert."

Even more than providing music that's structurally similar to what a particular individual enjoys, however, the Internet allows listeners to find their music "soul mate," another individual with a strikingly similar taste in music. This connection can be a potential source of many new musical acquisitions, because the likelihood of the soul mate's suggestions being useful is very high—much higher than the suggestions of any "expert." iTunes, for example, provides the opportunity to view playlists of potential music soul mates. With innovations such as this, the process is no longer passive: The listener is actively and fruitfully searching for music that will resonate.

Wikipedia, the Internet-based encyclopedia, is another entity that acquires strength as participation increases. What's remarkable about Wikipedia, which has grown steadily by receiving input from many "nonexpert" sources, is not how vast it has become, but how accurate. This is a proven entity that has acquired not only breadth but precision without the need to identify or rely on "experts." "Expertise," in this sphere, arises from cumulative experience rather than from one very competent person's experience.

Could we apply Internet music's concepts of soul mates and idea sharing and the music genome to the world of back pain? Could a database by and for back pain sufferers become as accurate and dense as Wikipedia? The answer to both questions is *yes*.

BACK PAIN RELIEF IN CYBERSPACE

What if an Internet-based database could collect all of the information related to your particular pain situation? This would include where the pain is, what positions make it worse, the duration of the pain, your age group, etc. It would also include the treatments that you've had so far and the results of those treatments. Imagine that the database would include your MRI findings along with the results of any other tests you've had. The more data you could supply, the more accurate and individualized the picture of your particular back pain presentation would become. In addition to the attributes of your pain, this database would ideally include details of your general health.

A full picture of your individuality would require information about your exercise and dietary habits, your desired and actual activities of daily living, and perhaps even your VO_2 level, your body fat composition, and your muscular strength. This database could then put you in touch with another individual with a strikingly similar presentation. Wouldn't that patient's experience with treatments be a helpful guide to allow you to choose a treatment? You bet it would.

Do you remember that earlier in the book I suggested that the treatment that you get depends on whom you see rather than what condition you have? Identifying your back "niche" and connecting to a back "soul mate" would be a way to overcome this bias of treatment, tied to where you start. As the database increased in size, so would its utility.

The idea of a database being collected and then used to serve as a tool for decision making seems to fly in the face of conventional wisdom. After all, the gold standard for decision making is the prospective, randomized, double-blind study. There's a push now in healthcare to use evidence-based medicine—that is, medicine evaluated by that sort of gold-standard study—as a means to determine treatment. What this means is that if a study is designed in advance to look at a particular problem (prospective), and the subjects studied are randomly assigned to the different treatment options (randomized), and the evaluation is done so that the evaluator and the one being evaluated are both unaware of what treatment was given (double-blind), the study is given maximal influence in its role as a decision-making tool.

The problems with prospective, randomized, double-blind studies are manifold: These studies are expensive, slow in execution, and limited in scope; in addition, they often contain biases that limit their application or their ability to be generalized.

Furthermore, the application of these studies to an individual has traditionally been left to healthcare providers. This is analogous to allowing the DJ to select the music on the radio station. The interpretation of these studies by a healthcare provider, along with the subsequent application to a single patient, introduces personal bias that further weakens the power of the information. In addition, the distribution of research findings is slow. For example, there's widespread agreement among experts about specific treatments such as the use of beta blockers after a heart attack, and yet the distribution of beta blockers is inconsistent from one geographic area to another.

Let me give you another example of the difficulties that we face with evidence-based medicine. Let's say we want to construct a study to decide whether yoga is good for patients with back pain. Most providers and most patients today would probably guess that yoga is good. If we want the best in evidence-based medicine, though, we'll need to make our study prospective, randomized, double-blind, and placebo-controlled, and we'll throw in a nontreatment cohort to eliminate regression to the mean (introduced in chapter 2). This study would, of

Core Concept

I envision that medicine—the treatment of back pain, in particular—will evolve in such a way that the patient will take the driver's seat. Patients with back pain will first identify their "niche" back pain presentation and record it in the back pain database. For example, a patient might present with intermittent episodes of low back pain and with an MRI that shows a disc bulge at L4–L5 and having failed McKenzie physical therapy. He might have a sedentary job and an 18 percent body fat composition. (Of course, the list of attributes would be much more detailed than this.) The patient will then combine this information with his own research on the topic (from his online access to the literature) and be directed to the appropriate healthcare provider, based on a survey of his back soul mates (a survey which demonstrated that this particular starting point has yielded the best results for others).

This patient will come into the encounter with that healthcare provider with an improved understanding due to his research on the Internet. With the benefit of the Internet's vast pool of information, the patient's starting point and knowledge base have both been optimized prior to the consultation. The chosen healthcare provider, whose education and experience help him or her filter available information, will then use that expertise to further the patient's educational process. In this process, the database, the accumulated literature, the patient's perspective, and the expertise of an individual practitioner act cooperatively to help with the back pain.

This is cooperative learning and cooperative decision making. This forward-looking approach is far superior to the current pedagogy. It doesn't diminish the value and need for prospective, randomized, double-blind studies. In fact, it serves to define which such studies are appropriate. To return to my earlier metaphor, the future of medicine will put you in the driver's seat and it will put the provider in the passenger's seat—to help with navigation—with the ultimate intent of getting you out of the car.

course, be expensive and time-consuming in its execution and subsequent analysis.

What if the study concluded that yoga was *not* beneficial? Providers and patients alike would be surprised and ask questions. Was the yoga studied the same yoga that I espouse? Was the yoga studied even all the same yoga? Yoga comes in many flavors, after all. How about the instructors? Were they all doing yoga the same way? What were their qualifications and how was consistency enforced? How about the patients? Did they all have the same type of back pain? How was this controlled for? How about the benefits; how were those determined? Objectively or subjectively? You see, what started out as a simple question became incredibly complicated.

We could anticipate some of these questions and make the study extremely narrow. Only a specific type of yoga and a specific type of instructor and a specific type of patient would be studied. This would give us results that would be more applicable to these specifics, but then we'd have to repeat the study, again and again, to look at all the other types of back pain and types of yoga to be useful for the whole population. In other words, the more satisfactory the study is, the less sufficient the study is.

THE BENEFIT OF "REAL TIME"

With back pain, the outcomes that need to be compared are often subjective. "How do you feel on a scale from one to ten?" or "Are you improved?" are examples of subjective questions. These differ fundamentally from objective questions such as, "How many miles can you walk?" It has been shown that patients are often not well equipped to answer subjective questions about "how they're doing" by memory alone. Responses to this seemingly easy sort of question can vary depending on when it's asked and how the patient is feeling when asked.

This is likely because we're designed to forget pain (just as mothers are designed to forget about the pain of childbirth). In this capacity as well, technology may be able to help.

The now-ubiquitous smart phone provides a means for accumulating "real-time" information about well-being. After-the-fact answers about how much pain a subject had are far less revealing than a real-time account of continuous data acquisition that records activities and pain throughout the day. Just as tweeting may ultimately serve as a means to write tomorrow's history books, real-time data acquisition may help to provide less biased or editorialized information about treatment results.

Smart phones can be equipped with cameras, accelerometers, microphones, and location sensors that can passively accumulate data that's more objective than the patient can be (or is willing to be) about activity levels, time spent lying down, social interactions, and so on. A combination of reflective data along with real-time acquired data collected before and after treatments of all kinds would provide a much better rationale for treatment than is available today. In essence, we'd be taking the guesswork out of what *is* basically guesswork. This information could be used to enrich the back genome database.

In the new medical world I envision, each person's back niche will be continually supplemented and refined by this combination of actively and passively acquired real-time data. This updating provides an alternative, more objective type of self-analysis (as opposed to self-reflection, psychotherapy, or reflective insight). For example, rather than deciding that one has "chronic back pain," an individual may find it more informative (or alternatively informative) to quantify the times in a day that the back pain prevents or impairs an activity of daily living, and to what degree.

Similarly, it may be helpful to quantify how often one takes pain medication, or how many days one misses from work, or when one's mood declines. This type of data acquisition has been used to answer questions such as whether a person is more productive with an extra hour of sleep or with an extra cup of coffee. On the surface, this is an easy question, but when we try to answer it, we realize that it's quite difficult. The correct answer requires the integration of large amounts of data and a definition of what "productive" means. When we're forced to define "productive" and accumulate evidence of productivity accurately, the answer to this question becomes much more meaningful. You can also see that a review of continuous data acquisition would better answer that type of question for *you*, specifically, than would a prospective, randomized, double-blind study done on a large population of other people.

SUPPLEMENTING THE BACK GENOME

Earlier I suggested that the development of a niche back pain presentation would be supplemented with access to the literature. It's not reasonable to expect you, a layperson, to be able to understand the literature well enough to apply it to your own situation. In fact, application of these studies to individual cases is difficult for me as an experienced healthcare provider, because there are always subtleties and nuances to incorporate into the decision process. The Internet is full of uncensored information, much of which is inaccurate. In addition, many studies are published and then either fade from use or are contradicted. Why do certain "great ideas" fail to get replicated or simply disappear? It's likely related to publication bias (an attraction to novel trends), the pervasive conflict of interest in our current literature (the studies having been funded or conducted by those with a financial interest in the product being studied), and, of course, the ability of humans to self-deceive.

Finally, it has been shown that many studies in the spine literature are written at a level that's simply not accessible to most patients with back pain. In one study, a program was used to assess the language in some of the more common spine-oriented websites. While it's generally recommended that studies or articles aimed at the public should be at a sixth-grade reading level, this study showed that spine information was often presented at a much higher level and suggested a pervasive disconnect to the majority of patients who look up medical information on the Internet for personal educational purposes.[2]

At this time, more than 50 percent of patients take the initiative of accessing medical literature on their own, with the number growing quickly. The above-cited inherent limitations that prevent you from fully appreciating the vast body of literature are fortuitous for me: I still have a job, and that job is to teach you, to guide you in your learning, and to help you make the best choices by applying the literature to your specific case.

POCKET THIS PARADOX

In an earlier chapter, I recommended seeing a specialist early in the course of back pain. This is unconventional, because it advises doing something that's not cost-effective and not practical. A database such as I have described, however, shortcuts the entire triage part of the healthcare system. You're not only starting with an expert, you're starting with *the most appropriate* expert. In addition, you're starting from a more educated position. Time spent with the expert is now a high-level educational session and a fine-tuning, rather than a rudimentary encounter. And, just to be clear, when I say "expert," I'm not necessarily referring to a neurosurgeon. An expert is the one whose qualifications and practices/techniques are best suited for the individual patient's back niche. That may be a physical therapist, a surgeon, a massage therapist, an acupuncturist, a mattress salesperson . . .

How will this new medical configuration affect the providers? We'll be seeing more "appropriate" patients, for starters, our competition having become *similar* providers, not *all* providers. As a surgeon, for example, I will undoubtedly see more patients with severe spinal stenosis and fewer with nonspecific back pain. I will react to this more appropriate distribution of patients by honing my surgical skills and improving my outcomes, because this will ultimately encourage additional patients to see me. I will design prospective, randomized, double-blind studies that are appropriately specific within my "narrowed" exposure to patients, making those studies more powerful and predictive than today's broad studies.

Many of the limitations in the current system are systemic in nature and inherently embedded. Some of these limitations are not going to change:

1. The minds of both providers and patients alike are inherently biased.

2. New knowledge takes time to disperse.

3. Ideal studies are expensive and slow in execution.

4. Healthcare is too expensive.

5. Providers are affected by how they're paid.

Despite these givens, I see a future that can fix back pain, and it lies in the back genome. Sure, the project will have its kinks, but what could be worse than where we are now? A bunch of mismatched patients and doctors, anxious about pain, addicted to prescription drugs, overspending on useless screening tests and therapies, collecting disability checks in the absence of true disability, litigiously protecting themselves from misdiagnosis (or, worse, no diagnosis), and overwrought with preconceived misconceptions, lies, and influences of culture and others.

We can reestablish our relationship and find synchronicity again, with patients empowered, educated, attuned to the mysteries of medicine, and physically strengthened, and doctors focused on fine-tuning the diagnosis and treatment—and then exiting the scene.

The back genome can do this, and more.

The Gist

- The future of medicine will put you in the driver's seat of back pain diagnostics, management, and treatment.

- Technology, as well as the changing definition of the word *expert,* will enable you to identify and access your back pain "soul mate" on the Internet. This connection will be vital in helping you choose an appropriate starting point for your evaluation, thereby maximizing the efficacy of your treatment.

ACKNOWLEDGMENTS

||||||||||||||||||||||||||||||||||||||||||||||||||||||||

I'd like to thank:

My father and mother, who taught me, by example, the importance of honesty and how to think for myself.

Cathy, my live-in editor—the real writer in our house.

John, Ed, Bruce, and Carlos, with whom I delightedly debated philosophy and learned how to think.

Roy, Arni, Dante, Ari, and Bernie, together with whom I learned to do spine surgery, had a great time, and formed great friendships.

Michele, Elsa, Miles, Nancy, and Francesca, who were invaluable in writing this book.

Phil, who taught me the art of kettlebells.

Matt, Domenick, and Beth, who taught me how a trained hand can heal.

Jerry, Brian, Dave, Lori, Matt, and Trella, for the photos, and Larissa, for the illustrations.

My patients, from whom I manage to learn more than I can teach.

NOTES
||||||||||||||||||

Introduction: How I Discovered the Hidden Core

1. Stuart McGill, *Ultimate Back Fitness and Performance* (Waterloo, Ontario: Wabuno, 2004), 16–17.

Chapter 1: The Brain and the Spine

1. E. Bennett, M. Diamond, D. Krech, and M. Rosenzweig, "Chemical and Anatomical Plasticity of the Brain," *Science* 164 (1964): 610–19.

2. Nassim Taleb, *Antifragile: Things That Gain from Disorder* (New York: Random House, 2012).

3. This widely quoted passage is from Nietzsche's *Twilight of the Idols*, published in 1889.

4. Richard Dawkins, *The Selfish Gene* (London: Oxford Univ. Press, 1976).

5. Norman Doidge, *The Brain That Changes Itself* (New York: Penguin, 2007).

6. B. Marcus et al., "Self-Efficacy and the Stages of Exercise Behavior Change," *Research Quarterly for Exercise and Sport* 63, no. 1 (Mar. 1992): 60–66.

7. Walter Bortz, *Next Medicine: The Science and Civics of Health* (New York: Oxford Univ. Press, 2011), 134.

8. This concept was put forward in Kierkegaard's *Concluding Unscientific Postscript to Philosophical Fragments*, published in 1846.

9. S. Gwilym et al., "Thalamic Atrophy Associated with Painful Osteoarthritis of the Hip Is Reversible After Arthroplasty: A Longitudinal Voxel-Based Morphometric Study," *Arthritis and Rheumatism* 62, no. 10 (2010): 2930–40.

10. G. Rizzolatti et al., "Mirror Neurons and Their Clinical Relevance," *Spine* 5 (2009): 24–34.

11. Bortz, *Next Medicine.*

12. John Ratey, *Spark: The Revolutionary New Science of Exercise and the Brain* (New York: Little, Brown, 2008).

Chapter 2: Pain

1. P. Kortebein et al., "Effect of 10 Days of Bed Rest on Skeletal Muscle in Healthy Older Adults," *Journal of the American Medical Association* 297 (2007): 1772–74.

2. T. Giesecke et al., "Evidence of Augmented Central Pain Processing in Idiopathic Chronic Low Back Pain," *Arthritis and Rheumatism* 50, no. 2 (2004): 613–23; P. Wood, "Variations in Brain Gray Matter Associated with Chronic Pain," *Current Rheumatology Reports* 12, no. 6 (2010): 462–69; M. Baliki et al., "Brain Morphological Signatures for Chronic Pain," *PLOS One* 6, no. 10 (2011): e26010.

3. Patrick Wall, *Pain: The Science of Suffering* (New York: Columbia Univ. Press, 2000).

4. Margaret Talbot, "The Placebo Prescription," *New York Times Magazine,* Jan. 9, 2000.

5. L. Cobb et al., "An Evaluation of Internal-Mammary-Artery Ligation by a Double-Blind Technic, *New England Journal of Medicine* 260 (May 28, 1959): 1115–18.

6. G. Crombez et al., "Pain-Related Fear Is More Disabling Than Pain Itself: Evidence on the Role of Pain-Related Fear in Chronic Back Pain Disability," *Pain* 80 (Mar. 1999): 329–39.

7. Nortin Hadler, *Stabbed in the Back: Confronting Back Pain in an Overtreated Society* (Chapel Hill: Univ. of North Carolina Press, 2009).

8. J. Katz, "Lumbar Disc Disorders and Low-Back Pain: Socioeconomic Factors and Consequences," *Journal of Bone and Joint Surgery (American)* 88, suppl. 2 (2006): 21–24.

9. Gordon Waddell, *The Back Pain Revolution,* 2nd ed. (London: Elsevier, 2004).

10. P. Kjaer et al., "Magnetic Resonance Imaging and Low Back Pain in Adults: A Diagnostic Imaging Study of 40-Year-Old Men and Women," *Spine* 30 (2005): 1173–80.

11. This passage is from Nietzche's *The Will to Power: A New Translation,* translated by Walter Kaufmann and R. J. Hollingdale, edited by Walter Kaufmann, published in 1967.

12. T. Videman et al., "Challenging the Cumulative Injury Model: Positive Effects of Greater Body Mass on Disc Degeneration," *The Spine Journal* 10, no. 1 (Jan. 2010): 26–31.

13. H. De Vries et al., "Staying at Work with Chronic Nonspecific Musculoskeletal Pain: A Qualitative Study of Workers' Experiences," *BMC Musculoskeletal Disorders* 12 (2011): 126; S. Dean et al., "Rural Workers' Experience of Low Back Pain: Exploring Why They Continue to Work," *Journal of Occupational Rehabilitation* 21 (2011): 395–409.

Chapter 3: The Anomaly and Anatomy of the Back

1. Andry Vleeming, *Movement, Stability, and Lumbopelvic Pain* (London: Churchill Livingstone, 2007).

2. Jim Johnson, *The Multifidus Back Pain Solution: Simple Exercises That Target the Muscles That Count* (Oakland: New Harbinger, 2002).

3. Jonathan FitzGordon, *Psoas Release Party! Release Your Body from Chronic Pain and Discomfort* (CreateSpace, 2013).

4. The two quotes that follow are from Frankl's *Man's Search for Meaning,* published in 1946.

Chapter 4: The Hidden Core Workout

1. Mark Sisson, *The Primal Blueprint: Reprogram Your Genes for Effortless Weight Loss, Vibrant Health, and Boundless Energy* (Philadelphia: Primal Nutrition, 2012).

2. Pavel Tsatsouline, *Enter the Kettlebell! Strength Secret of the Soviet Supermen* (St. Paul: Dragon Door Publications, 2006).

3. K. Jay et al., "Effects of Kettlebell Training on Postural Coordination and Jump Performance: A Randomized Controlled Trial," *Journal of Strength and Conditioning Research* 24, no. 3 (Mar. 2010): 730–36.

4. K. Jay, "Kettlebell Training for Musculoskeletal and Cardiovascular Health: A Randomized Controlled Trial," *Scandinavian Journal of Work, Environment, and Health* 37, no. 3 (May 2011): 196–203.

5. This concept is developed in Sartre's 1946 essay "Existentialism as a Humanism."

6. P. Hendrick et al., "The Effectiveness of Walking as an Intervention for Low Back Pain: A Systematic Review," *European Spine Journal* 25, no. 7 (2010): 79.

7. M. Terti, *American Journal of Sport Medicine* 18, no. 2 (1990): 206–8.

8. Christopher McDougall, *Born to Run: A Hidden Tribe, Superathletes, and the Greatest Race the World Has Never Seen* (New York: Random House, 2011); R. Hersher, "Perfect Landing: Study Finds Barefoot Runners Have Less Foot Stress Than Shod Ones," *Harvard Gazette*, Jan. 27, 2010; D. Lieberman et al., "Foot Strike Patterns and Collision Forces in Habitually Barefoot Versus Shod Runners," *Nature* 463 (2010): 531–35.

Chapter 5: Diagnosis

1. M. Underwood, "Diagnosing Acute Nonspecific Low Back Pain: Time to Lower the Red Flags?" *Arthritis and Rheumatism R_x* 60, no. 10 (Oct. 2009): 2855–57.

2. Craig Liebenson, *Rehabilitation of the Spine: A Practitioner's Manual* (Philadelphia: Lippincott Williams & Wilkins, 2007).

3. R. Chou and P. Shekelle, "Will This Patient Develop Persistent Disabling Low Back Pain?," *Journal of the American Medical Association* 303 (2010): 1295–1302.

4. A. Filler et al., "Sciatica of Non-Disc Origin and Piriformis Syndrome," *Journal of Neurosurgery: Spine* 2 (2005): 99–115.

5. A. Burton et al. (on behalf of COST B13 Working Group 3), "European Guidelines for Prevention in Low Back Pain," sponsored by the European Commission, Research Directorate General, Department of Policy, Coordination, and Strategy; www.backpaineurope.org; 2004.

Chapter 6: The Nonsurgical Treatment of Back Pain

1. S. Iyengar, "When Choice Is Demotivating: Can One Desire Too Much of a Good Thing?" *Journal of Personality and Social Psychology* 79, no. 6 (Dec. 2000): 995–1006.

2. R. Chou et al., "Medications for Acute and Chronic Low Back Pain: A Review of the Evidence for an American Pain Society/American College of Physicians Clinical Practice Guideline," *Annals of Internal Medicine* 147 (2007): 505–14.

et al., "Safety and Efficacy of Chymopapain (Chymodiactin) in Herniated
s Pulposus with Sciatica: Results of a Randomized, Double-Blind Study,"
al of the American Medical Association 249, no. 18 (1983): 2489–94.

Field et al., "Preterm Infant Massage Therapy Research: A Review," *Infant Behavior and Development* 33, no. 2 (Apr. 2010): 115–24.

5. O. Airaksinen et al., "European Guidelines for the Management of Chronic Nonspecific Low Back Pain," *European Spine Journal* 15, suppl. 2 (2007): S192–300; A. Furlan et al., "Massage for Low Back Pain: A Systematic Review Within the Framework of the Cochrane Collaboration Back Review Group," *Spine* 27 (2002): 1896–1910.

6. P. Kortebein et al., "Effect of 10 Days of Bed Rest on Skeletal Muscle in Healthy Older Adults," *Journal of the American Medical Association* 297 (2007): 1772–74.

7. A. Furlan et al., "Acupuncture and Dry-Needling for Low Back Pain: An Updated Systematic Review Within the Framework of the Cochrane Collaboration," *Spine* 30 (2005): 944–63; B. Brinkhaus et al., "Acupuncture in Patients with Chronic Low Back Pain: A Randomized Controlled Trial," *Archives of Internal Medicine* 166 (2006): 450–57.

8. M. Vitiello et al., "Cognitive Behavioral Therapy for Insomnia Improves Sleep and Decreases Pain in Older Adults with Comorbid Insomnia and Osteoarthritis," *Journal of Clinical Sleep Medicine* 5, no. 4 (2009): 1–8.

9. S. French et al., "Superficial Heat or Cold for Low Back Pain," *Cochrane Database of Systematic Reviews* 1 (Jan. 2006): CD004750.

10. William Broad, *The Science of Yoga: The Risks and the Rewards* (New York: Simon & Schuster, 2012).

Chapter 7: Surgery

1. Jerome Groopman and Pamela Hartzband, *Your Medical Mind: How to Decide What Is Right for You* (New York: Penguin, 2012).

Chapter 8: The Back Genome

1. Chris Anderson, *The Long Tail: Why the Future of Business Is Selling Less of More* (New York: Hyperion, 2006).

2. M. Vives et al., "Readability of Spine-Related Patient Education Materials from Subspecialty Organization and Spine Practitioner Websites," *Spine* 34 (2009): 2826.

INDEX
|||||||||||||||||

Abdominal muscles, 6, 59–60, 68, 98–99
Active release therapy, 168, 169
Acupuncture, 172–173
Acute pain, 52–54
Adaptation, 24–26
Advanced core exercises, 116–119
Aerobic exercises, 25, 90
American Association of Neurological
    Surgeons, 196
American Medical Association, 179
Analgesics, 162
Andersen, Hans Christian, 55
Anderson, Chris, 215
Annular tear, 137
Annulus, 137
Anterior abdominal exercises, 68
Anterior core muscles, 97, 100, 105, 115
Anterior deeper muscles, 70
Anterior superficial muscles, 69–70
Antidepressants, 162–163
*Antifragile: Things That Gain from
    Disorder* (Taleb), 12
Antifragility, 12
Antiseizure medications, 163
Anxiety, 162
Apollo, 213
Arthritis
    of facet joints, 145, 148
    facet joints and development of, 144
    spinal stenosis and, 147
    use of nonsteroidal anti-inflammatories
        for, 160
Asclepius, 213

Asymmetric stress, 67
Autogenic training techniques, 175
Awareness, 61–63

Back anatomy
    anterior deeper muscles, 70
    anterior superficial muscles, 69
    hidden core, 70–82
    visible core, 69–70
Back-bending, 62, 65–66, 104
Back extension on a fitness ball, 111–112
Back genome, 214–217, 221, 222–223
Back muscles, 66, 97
Back pain. *See also* Pain
    atrophy of multifidus muscles and, 78
    caused by spinal stenosis, 149
    degenerative disc disease, 152–153
    diagnosing common types of,
        145–156
    diagnostic testing for, 130–132
    disability, 45–46
    as disease, 46–52
    due to pregnancy, 78
    emperor's new clothes and, 55
    exercises and, 214
    from facet joints, 143–145
    hamstring tightness and, 81
    from herniated disc, 77
    herniated discs and, 138
    with leg pain and herniated discs,
        139–142
    microdiscectomy for, 203–204
    motion and, 89

(continued)

al treatment of, 157–181

ght people with, 154–156

t of life, 13

istent, 67

phenomenon of Westernized
societies, 46

pinching capsule of facet joint as
source for, 77

piriformis syndrome, 150–151

postsurgical, 78

potential causes of, 84

prevailing notions of, 50

reality of, 124–127

sciatica and, 150

smiling and, 23

spinal instability, 153–154

spinal stenosis and, 145–149

spondylolisthesis and, 152

surgery success rate for, 197

treatment with narcotics, 161

use of acupuncture for, 172

work and, 50–52

yoga and, 180

Bacon, Francis, 8

Baggage handlers, 63

Balneotherapy, 179–180

Bandura, Albert, 15

Barefoot runners, 92

Barr, Joseph, 48

BDNF. *See* Brain-derived neurotrophic
factor (BDNF)

Behavioral therapy, 175

Bending, 61–68

Bent-over kettlebell row, 112–113

Biceps femoris muscle, 80

Bloodletting, 38

Born to Run (McDougall), 92

Bortz, Walter, 16

Brafman, Ori, 48

Brafman, Rom, 48

Brain
assuming responsibility for health
and, 16–18
complexity of, 21–22
development, 14
embodied cognition and, 19
executive function of, 22
exercises and growth of, 25
judicial function of, 22, 29–31, 56, 74
multitasking and, 41–42

pain and, 33–34
rewiring, 15
role in enabling health, 14–15
self-efficacy and, 15–16
spine and, 14
virtual, 20–23
virtual pain map in, 21–22

Brain-derived neurotrophic factor
(BDNF), 25

Burpee, 116–117, 120

Capsaicin cream, 180

Capsule, 76, 145

Central nervous system, 33

Cerebral cortex, 35

Chameleon effect, 48

Chest pain, study looking at treatment,
39

Chiropractic, 179

Chiropractors, 168, 190

Chronic pain, 52–54, 78

Chymopapain, 166

Cleaning out, 209

Cobb, Leonard, 39

Cognitive therapy, 31

Cold compresses, 177–178

Collaboration, 183

Collagen fibers, 172

Collagen fibrils, 172

Comparison treatment, 190

Complications, 198–199

Compresses, hot versus cold, 177–178

Compression, 48

Compression fractures, 167

Computed tomography (CT) scans, 167,
188

Connective tissue modeling, 167

Connective tissue therapies, 169–172

Consultation, 189

Cooperative decision making, 219

Core, 59

Core concepts
of chameleon effect, 48
core strengthening, 74
herniated discs, 137
of nature of perceptions, 20
role of multifidus muscles, 78

Core strength, 61

Core strengthening, 180

Counter-nutation, 66

Crunches, 68

CT scans. *See* Computed tomography (CT) scans

Daily activities, 198
Databases, 215–219
Dawkins, Richard, 14
DEA. *See* U.S. Drug Enforcement Administration
Deadlifts, 87, 106–107
Decision-making tools, 218, 219
Decompression, 208–209
Deep braces, front view of, 71
Deep breathing techniques, 175
Degenerative disc disease, 92, 152–153, 208
Dementia, 147
Dendrites, 25
Depression, 91
Dermatomes, 139, 141
Descartes, René, 7, 32
Desiccation, 135
Dextrose, 179
Diagnosis
   common types of back pain, 145–156
   current model of, 215
   disc problem, 134–143
   do-it-yourself, 132–156
   early education and, 126–127
   facet problem, 134–135, 143–145
   Internet-based research and, 215–216
   patient history and, 185
   piriformis syndrome, 150–151
   role of healthcare providers, 125
   second opinions, 186
   seeking, 121–124
   spondylolisthesis, 151–152
   use of magnetic resonance image for, 189
Diagnostic language, 48–49
Diminished cues of failure ingredient, 16
Disability, 45–46, 50
Disc bulge, 48, 137
Disc extrusion, 48
Disc herniation. *See* Herniated discs
Disclaimers, 93–94
Discogenic pain, 133–134
Discogram, 131, 164–165
Disc problem, 134–135
Disc protrusion, 137
Dorsal column stimulation, 165

Dorsal column stimulator, 35
Dumbbells, 87

Einstein, Albert, 193
Electromyography (EMG) tests, 77, 78
Embodied cognition, 19
EMG tests. *See* Electromyography (EMG) tests
"The Emperor's New Clothes" (Andersen), 55
Endogenous opiates, 161
Endorphins, 161
Endoscopes, 166, 203
Epidural fibrosis, 200–201
Epidural injection, 163
Epigenetics, 24
Epinephrine, 169
Epiphenomenon, 28–29, 56, 74, 84
Erector spinae muscles, 74, 112
Europe, 200
Evidence-based medicine, 218
Excessive sweating syndrome, 164
Executive function, 22
Exercise ball, 87
Exercises
   advanced core, 116–119
   anterior abdominal, 68
   back extension on a fitness ball, 111–112
   bent-over kettlebell row, 112–113
   Burpee, 116–117
   cognitive therapy and, 31
   dendritic sprouting and, 25
   front plank, 98–99
   functional, 105
   hamstring curl on the fitness ball, 109–110
   hip-hinging, 106
   to improve back pain from herniated disc, 77
   isometric anterior core, 98–99
   kettlebell, 87–89, 101–102, 106–107, 112–115, 117–119
   kneeling swimmer's stretch, 96–97
   manual therapy and, 172
   of motion, 84
   multifidus muscles and, 78
   muscles and, 171
   neurogenesis and, 25
   oblique V-up, 108
   oxytocin and, 169

(continued)
45
of, 26
nary treatment of back pain, 214
onin and, 25
e plank, 99–100
ymmorphosis and, 24–25
Turkish get-up, 117–119
warm-up, 94–97
yoga cat stretch, 94–96
External oblique muscles, 70, 99

Facet block, 131–132
Facet injection, 164
Facet joints, 76–77, 143–145, 148, 173, 204
Facetogenic pain, 133–134
Facet problem, 134–135
Fascia, 71, 74, 76, 77, 138
Fibrils, 172
Finland, 50
Fitness balls, 87, 109–110, 111–112
Flat back, 68
Flexibility, 180
Flexion, 143
Fluoroscopes, 163, 164, 167
Fluoroscopy, 131
Form, 61, 87–89
Fractures, 167
Frankl principle, 81
Frankl, Viktor, 81
Front plank exercise, 98–99
Functional exercises, 105
Fusion, 202, 205–208

Gate control theory of pain, 34–35, 165
Genome, 24
The Girl with the Dragon Tattoo (Larsson), 41
Gluteal muscles, 68, 79, 89, 104, 112
Gluteus maximus muscle, 68, 79
Gluteus medius muscle, 68, 79
Gluteus minimus muscle, 68, 79
Golf, 187
Good Morning Stretch, 102–104
Greek mythology, 213
The Gutenberg Galaxy (McLuhan), 215
Gymnasts, 91

Hamstring Curl on the Fitness Ball, 109–110

Hamstring muscles
exercises for, 104–105, 107, 109–110
flat back and, 68
Hidden Core Workout for, 63
kettlebell exercises for, 87
overview of, 80–81
Hands-on therapies
acupuncture, 172–173
McKenzie physical therapy, 173, 174, 175
muscle and connective tissue therapies, 169–172
for pain management, 167–174
Happiness, 23
Headaches, 47
Healing Back Pain: The Mind-Body Connection (Sarno), 36
Healthcare, 17
Healthcare providers, 218
Health promotion, 214
Heating, 130
Heel strike, 92
Hellerwork, 169
Herniated discs
back pain and, 77
diagnostic language and, 48–49
leg pain and, 138
lumbar traction therapy for, 174
McKenzie physical therapy for, 173
multifidus muscles and, 78
overview of, 138
sciatica and, 150
use of MRI for diagnosis of, 124, 128–129, 142
younger patients and, 135
Herniated lumbar discs, 203
Hidden core muscles, 59–60, 100
Hidden Core Workout
advanced core exercises, 116–119
breakdown of, 90
core strengthening and, 74
developing posterior chain of muscles in, 72
epiphenomenon and, 56
equipment needed for, 87
hip-hinging, 63
isometrics to movement in, 84
judicial function of brain and, 56
pain and, 54–56
painful stimulus and, 54
strengthening gluteal muscles, 79
week five, 111–113

week five recap, 113
week four, 106–110
week four recap, 110
week one, 94–99
week one recap, 97
week six, 114–115
week six recap, 120
week three, 101–105
week three recap, 105
week two, 98–100
week two recap, 100
yoga and, 180
High-speed precision drills, 203
Hip flexor muscles, 68
Hip-hinging, 62, 63, 65–66, 104, 106
Hippocrates of Cos, 91
Hippocratic Oath, 212
Holmes, Oliver Wendell, 38
Hormones, 169
Hot compresses, 177–178
Human genome project, 214
Hydrogen bonds, 172
Hygeia, 213
Hyperlordosis, 68
Hypertrophic spinal tissue, 208
Hypertrophy, 171

IGF-1. *See* Insulin-like growth factor
  (IGF-1)
Iliacus muscle, 68
Iliocostalis muscles, 74
Ilium bones, 152
Image-guided technology, 20
Imaging techniques, 175
Immobility, 84
Impingement, 48
Inactivity, 171
Independence, 16
Inflammation
  conventional view of, 12
  effects of dextrose on, 179
  herniated discs and, 140
  hot compresses and, 178
  medications that reduce, 160
  of nerve roots, 150
  painful stimulus and, 28
Injections
  discogram, 164–165
  epidural injection, 163
  facet injection, 164
  intra-articular injection, 164

for pain management, 163–165
  selective root block, 164
  sympathetic ganglion block, 164
Instability, 29, 153–154
Instinct, 158–159, 195
Insulin-like growth factor (IGF-1), 25
Insurance coverage
  acupuncture, 172
  for hands-on therapies, 168
Integrative therapies
  balneotherapy, 179–180
  capsaicin cream, 180
  for pain management, 178–180
  prolotherapy, 178–179
  willow bark, 180
Intensity, 42
Internal brace, 59–61, 70–73, 81
Internal oblique muscles, 70, 99
Internet-based research, 214, 215–216,
  219, 222–223
Intra-articular injection, 164
Intrathecal delivery, 165–166
Invasive diagnostic testing, 130–132
Invasive procedures
  decompression, 208–209
  dorsal column stimulation, 165
  fusion, 205–208
  intrathecal delivery, 165–166
  kyphoplasty, 167
  microdiscectomy, 203–205
  minimally, 167, 202–203
  for pain management, 165–167
  percutaneous discectomy, 166–167
  surgery of spine, 202–203
Isometric anterior core exercise, 98–99
Isometrics, 84
iTunes, 216

Janda, Vladimir, 68
Judicial function
  core strengthening and, 74
  defined, 22
  in Hidden Core Workout, 56
  pain and, 29–31, 84

Kettlebell deadlift, 106–107
Kettlebells
  exercises using, 87–89, 101–102,
    106–107, 112–115, 117–119
  overview of, 88
  use to overcome back pain, 3–4, 87–89

...t, 101–102
...ings, 87–89, 114–115, 120
...d principle, 18, 94
...ard, Søren, 7, 18
...ig effect, 29
...ing swimmer's stretch, 96–97
...hoplasty, 167
...yphotic back, 68–69

L2 Nerve root dermatome, 140
L2 Nerve root myotome, 140
L3 Nerve root dermatome, 140–141
L3 Nerve root myotome, 141
L4 nerve root dermatome, 142
L4 nerve root myotome, 142
L5 nerve root dermatome, 142
L5 nerve root myotome, 142
L5 nerve roots, 188
Laminectomy, 209
Laminotomy, 209
Larsson, Stieg, 41
Lateral core muscles, 100, 115
Lateral muscles, 70
Latissimus dorsi muscles, 72, 113
Leg pain
  with back pain, 134
  with back pain and herniated discs,
    139–142
  herniated discs and, 138
  magnetic resonance image for, 188
  microdiscectomy for, 203–204
  in spinal stenosis, 149
  spinal stenosis and, 149
  spondylolisthesis and, 152
  surgery success rate for, 197
  use of antidepressants for, 163
Lidocaine, 162
Lidoderm patch, 162
Lifting, 61
Ligamentum flavum, 143
Limbic system, 35
Live X-ray, 131
Longissimus muscles, 74
Longitudinal massage, 167
The Long Tail (Anderson), 215
Lordosis, 68, 104
Loupe, 203
Lower back muscles, 104
Lower cross syndrome, 68
Lumbar spine. See also Spine
  in flat back, 68

of forty-year-old, 49
hidden core muscles and, 78
magnetic resonance image for, 4, 189,
  207
psoas muscles and, 79
sacroiliac joint and, 152
spinal stenosis and, 146
surgery, 197
Lumbar traction therapy, 174
Lying down, 189

Magnetic resonance image (MRI)
  comparison treatment and, 191
  functional, 31, 39
  kyphoplasty, 167
  for leg pain, 188
  of lumbar spine, 4, 191
  McKenzie physical therapy and use of,
    173
  of multifidus muscles, 78
  of runners, 91
  traction therapy and use of, 174
  use for diagnosis of back pain,
    130–131, 189
  use for diagnosis of herniated disc,
    48–49, 124, 128–129, 142
  use of image-guided technology and,
    20
  use to determine cause of pain, 17, 28
Marx, Groucho, 29, 67
Maslow, Abraham, 122, 155
Massage, 130, 167
Mattress "therapy," 174–176
Maugham principle, 23, 93, 94
Maugham, Somerset, 23
Maximal strength, 85
McDougall, Christopher, 92
McKenzie physical therapy, 173, 174, 175,
  219
McKenzie, Robin, 173
McLuhan, Marshall, 215
Mechanical pain, 188
Medical literature, 222–223
Medications
  analgesics, 162
  antidepressants, 162–163
  antiseizure, 163
  muscle relaxants, 162
  narcotics, 160–162, 166
  nocebo effect and, 40–41
  nonsteroidal anti-inflammatories, 160

for pain management, 159–163
placebo effect, 35–39, 40
placebos and pain, 39–40
steroidal anti-inflammatories, 160
walking as an alternative to, 91
Memes, 14
Microdiscectomy, 166, 200, 203–205
Microscopes, 166, 203
Midline preservation, 209
Minimal access, 202–203
Minimally invasive surgery, 167, 202
Mirror neurons, 21
Misplaced spinal tissue, 208
Mixter, William, 48
Mood elevation, 180
Motion, 28, 89
Motor nerves, 33
Motor strip, 35
MRI. *See* Magnetic resonance image
  (MRI)
Multifidus muscles
  exercises for, 112, 113
  flat back and, 68
  herniated discs and, 130
  hidden core muscles and, 5, 74–78
  kyphotic back and, 69
  spinal stenosis and, 148
Multitasking, 41–42
Muscle relaxants, 162
Muscle relaxation techniques, 175
Muscles
  abdominal, 6, 59–60, 68
  anterior core, 97, 100, 105, 115
  anterior deeper, 70
  anterior superficial, 69–70
  back, 66
  beneficial effects of applying pressure
    to, 171
  biceps femoris, 80
  electromyography tests of, 77, 78
  erector spinae, 74, 112
  external oblique, 70, 99
  gluteal, 68, 79, 89, 104, 112
  hamstring, 63, 68, 80–81, 87–89,
    102–105, 107, 109–110
  hidden core, 5, 59–60
  hip flexor, 68
  hypertrophy, 171
  iliacus, 68
  iliocostalis, 74
  inactivity, 171

internal oblique, 70, 99
joints and, 171
lateral core, 100, 115
lateral muscles, 70
latissimus dorsi, 72, 113
longissimus, 74
lower back, 104
mass, 171
multifidus, 5, 68, 69, 74–78, 112, 113,
  138, 148
oblique, 104, 108, 113
pain fibers and, 170
pain management, 169–172
paraspinal, 97
pectoralis, 72
piriformis, 150
posterior core, 71, 74, 100, 111, 112
psoas, 79–80
psoas major, 68
quadratus lumborum, 79
quadriceps femoris, 73
rectus abdominis, 69–70, 108, 110
rectus femoris, 68
rhomboid, 68–69, 113
semimembranosus, 80
semitendinosus, 80
serratus anterior, 69, 72
six-pack abdominal, 59–60, 70
stretching and strengthening of the,
  84–85
striated, 170
that line and stabilize the spine, 170
transversalis abdominis, 6, 110
transversus abdominis, 70
trapezius, 69
Muscle spasms
  back pain and, 2
  cold compresses and, 177
  epiphenomenon and, 28–29, 84, 138
  muscle relaxants and, 162
  treatment of back pain and, 168
Muscle therapies, 169–172
Muscle tissue, 170
Musculature, 170
Myelin, 33
Myofascial release therapy, 169
Myotomes, 139

Narcotics, 160–162, 166
Neocortex, 22
Nerve roots, 139–142, 150, 200, 203

Nervous system, 33
Netherlands, 51
Neurogenesis, 25
Neuromuscular therapy, 169
Neurons, 21, 25
Neuropathy, 163
Neurosurgeons, 195
New Zealand, 51
Next Medicine (Bortz), 16
"Niche" cultural tastes, 215–216
Nietzsche, Friedrich, 7, 13, 49, 211
Nietzsche principle, 13, 85
Nocebo effect, 40–41
Nongymnasts, 91
Nonmechanical pain, 188
Nonsteroidal anti-inflammatories
    (NSAIDs), 160
Non-Westernized societies, 46
Norepinephrine, 162
Normal posture, 67
Novelty, 42
NSAIDs. *See* Nonsteroidal anti-
    inflammatories (NSAIDs)
Numbness, 139, 163
Nutation, 63–66

Obese patients, 68
Obesity, 91
Oblique muscles, 104, 108, 113
Oblique V-up, 108
Of Human Bondage (Maugham), 23
Older patients, 87, 144, 191–192
Opinions, 94
Osteopaths, 168
Osteoporosis, 167, 176–177
Overweight people, 88, 154–156
Oxytocin, 169

Pain. *See also* Back pain
    acute, 52–54
    from asymmetric stress, 67
    attributes of, 42
    brain and, 33–34
    chronic, 52–54
    diagnostic testing for provoking,
        131
    diagnostic testing for relieving,
        131–132
    distinction between disability and,
        45–46
    dualistic conception of, 32
    epiphenomenon of, 28–29
    facet-generated, 144
    gate control theory of, 34–35
    herniated discs as cause of, 138–142
    Hidden Core Workout and, 54–56
    intensity of, 42
    judicial function of brain and, 29–31
    localizing segment of pain generation,
        206
    mechanical, 188
    modern theory of, 32–33, 35
    motion and, 29
    natural control of, 161
    nocebo effect and, 40–41
    nonmechanical, 188
    nonspinal origins, 132–133
    novelty of, 42
    painful stimulus and, 27–28
    perceived threat of, 42–43
    perception of, 36–37
    placebo effect, 35–39
    placebos and, 39–40
    postoperative, 200
    purpose and priority of, 41–45
    sacroiliac joint, 152
    as somatic manifestation of repressed
        emotions, 36
    spinal origins, 132–133
    three-tiered causation of, 27–33
    tolerance for, 187
Pain fibers, 170
Painful stimulus, 27–28, 53, 54, 74, 84
Pain management
    hands-on therapies, 167–174
    hot versus cold compresses, 177–178
    injections, 163–165
    integrative therapies, 178–180
    invasive procedures, 165–167
    mattress "therapy," 174–176
    medications, 159–163
    muscle and connective tissue
        manipulation for, 170
Pain resolution, 197
Palmer, Daniel David, 179
Panacea, 213
Pandora's Box, 48
Paraspinal muscles, 97
Patient-driven care, 214
Patient history, 185, 188
Pectoralis muscles, 72
Peer examples ingredient, 16

Pelvis, 63, 66, 68, 72, 74, 152
Perceived threat, 42–43
Perceptions, 20
Percutaneous discectomy, 166–167
Peripheral nervous system, 33
Pessimism, 43
Phenotypic plasticity, 24
Physical therapists, 168
Physical therapy
  active role in healing and, 190
  for back pain, 31
  herniated discs and, 138, 143
  longitudinal massage, 167
  McKenzie physical therapy, 173
  for spinal stenosis, 149
  strengthening and stretching, 84
Pilates, 6
Piriformis muscle, 150
Piriformis syndrome, 150–151
Placebo effect
  acupuncture and, 173
  defined, 37
  overview of, 35–39
  percutaneous discectomy and, 166
Plantar fasciitis, 167
Posterior chain muscles, 71
Posterior core muscles, 71, 74, 100, 111, 112
Posterior longitudinal ligament, 143
Postoperative pain, 200
Postsurgical back pain, 78
Postural change, 28–29, 84, 138, 170
Posture
  common variants of, 67–69
  flat back, 68
  hyperlordosis, 68
  kettlebell exercises for, 87–89
  kyphotic back, 68–69
  normal, 67
  role of quadratus lumborum muscles, 79
  standing, 61, 145
  sway back, 67
  treatment to improve, 69
Pregnancy, 78, 152
Primal instincts, 86
Primed states, 43
Prolotherapy, 178–179
Prometheus, 48
Psoas major muscle, 68
Psoas muscles, 79–80

Qi, 172
Quadratus lumborum muscles, 79
Quadriceps femoris muscles, 73

Radiculopathy, 150
"Real-time" information, 220–222
Rectus abdominis muscles, 69, 70, 108, 110
Rectus femoris muscle, 68
Reflex sympathetic dystrophy syndrome, 164
Regression to the mean, 38
Relaxation techniques, 175, 180
Research, 214
Responsibility, 16–18, 185, 214
Rhomboid muscles, 68–69, 113
Role models ingredient, 16
Rolfing, 168, 169, 172
Roman chair, 2, 5
Runners, 91, 92
Running, 90–92

S1 nerve root dermatome, 142
S1 nerve root myotome, 142
Sacroiliac joint, 63–64, 66, 72, 77
Sacroiliac joint pain, 152
Sacrum, 63, 66, 79, 152
Salicylic acid, 180
Sarno, John, 36–37
Sartre, Jean-Paul, 7, 91
Sartre principle, 91
Scapula stabilizers, 68
Scar tissue, 167–168, 200–201
Sciatica, 150
Sciatic nerve, 150
Second opinions, 186, 199–200
Seizure disorders, 163
Selective root block, 164
Self-efficacy, 15–16, 180
Self-empowerment, 185
Self-labeled behaviors, 91
Semimembranosus muscle, 80
Semitendinosus muscle, 80
Sensory nerves, 33
Sequestered disc, 137
Serotonin, 25, 162
Serratus anterior muscles, 69, 72
Shod runners, 92
Shopping cart sign, 149
Side plank exercise, 99–100
SI joint. *See* Sacroiliac joint
Six-pack abdominal muscles, 59–60, 70

Sleep, 175, 176
Sleep disturbances, 91
Small steps ingredient, 16
Smart phones, 214, 221
Smiling, 23
Social persuasion ingredient, 16
Soft-tissue pain, 28–29
Somatic states, 43
Spinal column, 170
Spinal cord, 162, 165
Spinal-derived pain, 132–134
Spinal instability, 153–154
Spinalis muscles, 74
Spinal stenosis, 145–149, 192
Spinal tissue, 208
Spine. *See also* Lumbar spine
  back-bending and, 65–66
  brain and, 14
  core strengthening and, 74
  discs and, 135
  of female gymnasts, 91
  of female nongymnasts, 91
  internal brace and, 72
  kettlebell exercises, 89
  muscles that line and stabilize, 170
  posterior core muscles and, 74–77
  running and, 92
  sacrum of, 63
  shopping cart and, 149
  S-shaped curve of, 67
  thoracic, 68
  tightening of fascia and, 71–72
Spinous process, 76–77
Spondylolisthesis, 4, 78, 151–152, 154
Stabilizer effect, 72
Standing, 61, 145
Standing Hamstring Stretch, 102–104
Steroidal anti-inflammatories, 160
Strengthening, 84–85, 100, 105
Stress
  asymmetric, 67
  conventional view of, 12
  exercises and, 24
  spinal column and, 170–171
Stretching, 84–85, 105, 130
Striated muscle, 170
Stronger-than-average men, 87
Structural integration therapy, 169
Success rates
  fusion, 208
  for surgery, 197

Sun Tzu, 121
Superficial braces, front view of, 71
Surgeons
  choosing, 195–196
  external biases of, 197
  invasive pain management procedures
    and, 165
  natural history of patient's problem
    and, 198
  second opinions, 199–200
Surgery
  choosing back surgeon, 195–196
  complications, 198–199
  considerations when deciding on,
    196–199
  contemplating, 193–194
  for herniated discs, 142
  hypothetical considerations,
    185–193
  individualized decisions for, 194
  negative perception of, 193–194
  normal nerve roots and, 140
  postoperative period, 200–201
  scar tissue, 200–201
  second opinions, 199–200
  spinal instability, 154
  for spinal stenosis, 146–147, 148, 149,
    192
  success rate, 197
Sway back, 67, 68
*Sway: The Irresistible Pull of Irrational
  Behavior* (Brafman & Brafman), 48
Swinging exercises, 88
Symmorphosis, 24–25
Sympathetic ganglion block, 164
Sympathetic system, 164
Synovial fluid, 144, 145
Synovium, 144, 145
System-based software, 215

Taleb, Nassim, 12
Technology
  Internet-based research and, 214,
    215–216, 219, 222–223
  "real-time" information and,
    220–222
  smart phones, 214, 221
Temperature, 164
Terminology, 48
Thalamus, 35
Therapy, 190

Therapy programs, 84
Thixotropy, 172
Thoracic spine, 68
Thoracolumbar fascia, 76
Tolerance, 187
Transversalis abdominis muscles, 6, 110
Transversalis fascia, 77
Transversus abdominis muscles, 6, 70
Trapezius muscle, 69
Turkish get-up, 117–119, 120

Unroofing, 209
U.S. Drug Enforcement Administration, 160

Vascular endothelial growth factor (VEGF), 25
Vasodilatation, 164
VAX-D. *See* Vertebral axial decompression (VAX-D)
VEGF. *See* Vascular endothelial growth factor (VEGF)
Vertebral axial decompression (VAX-D), 174

Virtual pain map, 21–22
Voltaire, 17

Walking, 90–92, 147
Warm-up exercises, 94–97
Weaker-than-average men, 87
Weight lifters, 61, 63
Westernized societies, 46
Wikipedia, 216
Willow bark, 180
Women, 87
Work, 50–52

X-rays, 166, 167, 207

Yellow ligament, 143
Yin and yang, 172
Yoga
    back twist, 104–105
    cat stretch, 94–96
    proposed study of, 218–220
    as treatment for back pain, 180
YouTube, 87

Zygapophyseal joint, 143

ABOUT THE AUTHOR

IIIIIIIIIIIIIIIIIIIIIIIIIIIIIIIIIIIIIIIIIIIIIIIIIIIII

Patrick Roth, M.D., is the chairman of the Department of Neurosurgery at Hackensack University Medical Center and the director of the Hackensack neurosurgical residency program. He has authored numerous publications related to the spine and has been perennially included in the Castle and Connolly Top Doctors listing, as well as in *New York* magazine's Best Doctors issue and *Inside Jersey*'s Top Doctors listing. His areas of focus include minimally invasive spinal surgery, rehabilitation of back pain, and exercise and diet. He lives in northern New Jersey with his wife and two children.

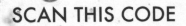

SCAN THIS CODE

WITH YOUR SMARTPHONE TO BE LINKED TO
THE BONUS MATERIALS FOR

THE END OF BACK PAIN

on the Elixir website,
where you can also find information about other
healthy living books and related materials.

YOU CAN ALSO TEXT

BACK to READIT (732348)

to be sent a link to the Elixir website.

 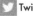